Aerobic Dance for Health and Fitness

Aerobic Dance for Health and Fitness

Lorna Francis
San Diego State University

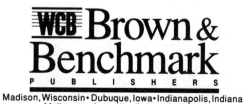

WCB Brown & Benchmark
PUBLISHERS

Madison, Wisconsin • Dubuque, Iowa • Indianapolis, Indiana
Melbourne, Australia • Oxford, England

Book Team

Editor *Chris Rogers*
Production Editor *Jayne Klein*

Brown & Benchmark

A Division of Wm. C. Brown Communications, Inc.

Vice President and General Manager *Thomas E. Doran*
Executive Managing Editor *Ed Bartell*
Executive Editor *Edgar J. Laube*
Director of Marketing *Kathy Law Laube*
National Sales Manager *Eric Ziegler*
Marketing Manager *Pamela Cooper*
Advertising Manager *Jodi Rymer*
Managing Editor, Production *Colleen A. Yonda*
Manager of Visuals and Design *Faye M. Schilling*

Production Editorial Manager *Vickie Putman Caughron*
Publishing Services Manager *Karen J. Slaght*
Permissions/Records Manager *Connie Allendorf*

Wm. C. Brown Communications, Inc.

Chairman Emeritus *Wm. C. Brown*
Chairman and Chief Executive Officer *Mark C. Falb*
President and Chief Operating Officer *G. Franklin Lewis*
Corporate Vice President, Operations *Beverly Kolz*
Corporate Vice President, President of WCB Manufacturing *Roger Meyer*

Cover and interior design by Matthew Doherty Design

Cover photo by Globus Studios, Inc.

Copyedited by Judy Lary

To my husband, Peter, and my children, Cameron and Ashley.

Contents

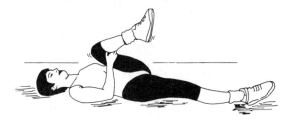

4 FLEXIBILITY AND STRETCHING   27

5 MUSCULAR STRENGTH AND ENDURANCE   50

Preface

Aerobic dance is a constantly changing fitness activity that continues to attract millions of participants each year. New advances in aerobic dance can be attributed to current scientific research and to the creative imaginations of dance exercise instructors. To help you develop a safe and effective fitness program, this book will familiarize you with the latest information about aerobic dance and exercise techniques.

Each chapter in the book begins with a short true/false quiz to test your knowledge of important fitness concepts. Common exercise myths are explored, and valuable fitness assessment tests are provided to determine your current level of physical fitness. Tips are offered to help you select the right aerobic dance program and to assist you in setting personal exercise and nutritional goals. Proper and improper exercises are illustrated, as well as common movement patterns used in aerobic dance choreography. In addition, sample exercise and aerobic dance routines are presented throughout the book.

Unique features of this book include the use of rubber bands and the introduction of interval and circuit training. Rubber bands provide the necessary resistance for enhancing muscular strength; interval and circuit training offer enjoyable alternatives to continuous forms of aerobic exercise. The book concludes with valuable information for helping you to manage your weight and for recognizing and preventing common aerobic dance injuries.

About the Author

Lorna Francis has been involved in the fitness industry since receiving her bachelor's degree in physical education from Iowa State University in 1976. While teaching exercise classes for both the university and the community, she completed a master's degree in physical education from Iowa State University. Combining her interest in sport and media, she obtained a doctorate in telecommunications and film from the University of Oregon.

Certified by ACE (the American Council on Exercise), Dr. Francis has taught at Iowa State University and the University of Oregon and is currently an assistant professor in the department of physical education at San Diego State University. She was chair of the San Diego Dance for Heart Committee (1985–1986), chair of the ACE Exam Committee on Standards and Certification in Dance Exercise (1989–1991), and a member of the board of directors for the Japan Aerobic Fitness Association (1989–1990).

Based on many years of teaching experience, research, and continuing education, Dr. Francis is internationally recognized for her practical, safe, and enjoyable approach to exercise. Over the years, Dr. Francis has developed a number of innovative programs for the fitness industry, including the Pre-Aerobic Program (exercise for deconditioned populations), BodyCheck (a practical system for evaluating health and fitness), and MIA (Moderate-Impact Aerobics).

Dr. Francis travels throughout the United States and the world giving lectures and workshops on the scientific and practical aspects of various fitness activities. She is a frequent contributor to fitness publications such as *Shape, Self,* and *IDEA Today*. Dr. Francis is co-author of the book, *If It Hurts, Don't Do It* (Prima Publisher, 1988).

Dr. Francis has served as exercise safety consultant on a number of videotapes, including *The Balanced Fitness Workout* (American College of Obstetricians and Gynecologists), *The BodyBand Workout* (American Academy of Family Physicians), *Teen Workout* (Field Productions), and *Introduction to Step Reebok* (Reebok International). She has appeared in two videotapes: *Injury Prevention through Fitness Assessment* and

Exercise Analysis: The E.S.P. System. As a current member of the Step Reebok Development Team, Dr. Francis conducts step-training research, develops new step-training programs, and writes instructor manuals.

In 1987, Dr. Francis was co-recipient of the IDEA (International Dance Exercise Association) Research Award for her work on a number of well-publicized research projects that examined the potential causes of fitness-related injuries. She was also co-recipient of the 1989 IDEA Lifetime Achievement Award in recognition of her service to the fitness industry.

Dr. Francis has appeared on national television, including NBC's "Today" show and ESPN's "Body Shaping," and she has been interviewed in magazines and newspapers such as *People, The National Enquirer, USA Today, Redbook, Shape, Self,* and *Vogue.*

1 *Staying Healthy and Fit*

TEST YOUR KNOWLEDGE

Answer true or false to the following statements:

1. The United States is currently experiencing a fitness boom.   True   False

   Answer: False. Although more people exercise today compared to twenty years ago, less than 20 percent of the adult American population exercise regularly enough to gain significant health benefits.

2. Of those who join a formal exercise program, at least half will drop out within the first year.   True   False

   Answer: True. Fifty to sixty percent will drop out within the first six months to a year.

3. High cholesterol levels and high blood pressure are greater risks factors for developing coronary heart disease than is inactivity.   True   False

   Answer: False. Researchers have recently found that sedentary behavior is as much a risk factor for heart disease as are high cholesterol and high blood pressure.

4. Exercise can increase your lifespan.   True   False

   Answer: True. Moderate levels of exercise can increase life expectancy.

How Fit Are Americans?

Although the media have led us to believe that Americans are in the midst of a fitness boom, recent statistics do not support this claim. It may be true that many more people exercise today compared to twenty years ago, but fewer than 20 percent of the adult American population exercise regularly enough to gain significant health benefits. Within six months to a year, 50 to 60 percent of those who join an exercise program drop out. What is even more alarming is that over 40 percent of the adult population do absolutely no exercise at all.

According to the Centers for Disease Control, inactivity as indicated by a sedentary life-style is as much a risk factor for coronary heart disease as is a high cholesterol level, high blood pressure, or smoking. In fact, the percentage of sedentary individuals in the United States exceeds the total percentage of Americans who have high cholesterol levels, who have high blood pressure, and who smoke a pack of cigarettes a day.

Fortunately, regular exercise can substantially reduce the risk of developing coronary heart disease, the number-one killer in the United States. Researchers have found that moderate levels of exercise, including activities such as walking, stair climbing, and sports play, can increase life expectancy. These findings are particularly important because they suggest that exercise does not have to be extremely vigorous to produce health benefits.

Developing Health-Related Fitness

To comfortably meet the demands of daily living, your body requires a minimal level of health-related fitness. A sound aerobic dance class will incorporate exercises and activities that address all components of health-related fitness, including cardiovascular endurance, body composition, muscular strength, muscular endurance, and flexibility.

Cardiovascular Endurance (Also Called Cardiorespiratory Endurance or Aerobic Fitness): Aerobic activities such as aerobic dance strengthen the cardiovascular system by improving the ability of the heart and lungs to deliver oxygen to the working muscles during sustained movement. Enhanced aerobic fitness allows you to perform more physical work with less fatigue and reduces your risk of developing coronary heart disease.

Body Composition: Regular participation in aerobic dance improves your body composition, which is the ratio of body fat to lean body weight (body weight that does not include fat). A reduction in total body fat not only improves your appearance but also decreases your chances of developing cardiovascular disease.

Muscular Strength: Muscular strength is the maximum amount of force that your muscles can exert against resistance. The strength segment of an aerobic dance class enhances your exercise performance, reduces the likelihood of sustaining injury by helping you maintain proper body mechanics and posture, and improves your appearance by developing greater muscle definition.

Muscular Endurance: The ability of your muscles to contract repeatedly against resistance over time requires muscular endurance. Aerobic dance will enhance your muscular endurance, allowing you to perform daily tasks for longer periods of time with less fatigue.

Flexibility: Flexibility describes the amount of movement possible at a joint. Maintaining an appropriate level of flexibility will allow you to reach and bend farther when necessary and help you to maintain good spinal alignment, which reduces the risk of developing common aches and pains such as back, neck, and shoulder discomfort.

Keep in mind that no single component of health-related fitness is more important than another. Each contributes to your total well-being.

Balancing Your Workouts

To improve or maintain health-related fitness, your workouts must be carefully balanced. Because all components of fitness are important for maintaining good health, your exercise program should include strength and flexibility exercises as well as aerobic activities.

You must also balance the activities and exercises within each component of fitness. For example, your strength program should include complementary exercises that strengthen muscles on both sides of the joint in order to minimize muscle imbalances. Similarly, you may choose to participate in several complementary aerobic activities to help balance the mechanical stress characteristic of each physical activity.

Basic Exercise Principles

Whether your workouts involve stretching, strengthening, or aerobic activity, the principles of overload, progression, reversibility, and specificity apply to all forms of exercise.

Overload: To gain various health benefits, your heart, lungs, and muscles must be challenged beyond the workload they are accustomed to performing. If the workload is too easy, you will not improve specific components of health-related fitness.

Progression: To allow your body adequate time to adapt to the new stresses of physical activity, you must gradually and systematically increase the amount of exercise. Exercising too fast, too often, or too hard too soon will increase your risk of injury.

Reversibility: Health benefits gained from exercise will be maintained only as long as you continue to exercise. When you stop exercising, you gradually lose the benefits you acquired from being physically active.

Specificity: The health benefits gained from exercise are specific to the type of activity in which you participate. For example, if you are enrolled in a yoga class, you can expect to increase your flexibility but you are not likely to improve your muscular strength or aerobic fitness. If you want to be a stronger runner, you must target and strengthen the specific muscles involved in the mechanics of running.

KEY POINTS IN CHAPTER 1

1. Regular participation in aerobic dance will help you improve all components of health-related fitness, including cardiovascular endurance, body composition, flexibility, muscular strength, and muscular endurance.

2. Improvements in cardiovascular endurance and body composition can significantly reduce your risk of developing heart disease, the number one killer in the United States.

3. Increased cardiovascular and muscular endurance will allow you to perform daily tasks, sports, and exercises for longer periods of time with less fatigue.

4. Enhanced muscular strength will improve your physical appearance and body mechanics.

5. Improved flexibility can improve your exercise performance and reduce your risk of developing common ailments such as low back pain.

6. Your aerobic dance program should be carefully balanced to include exercises for each component of health-related fitness.

7. When designing an exercise program, keep in mind the principles of overload, progression, reversibility, and specificity.

2 How Fit Are You?

TEST YOUR KNOWLEDGE

Answer true or false to the following statements:

1. Most people will experience some form of back pain during their adult years.　　True　　False

   Answer: True. Eight out of ten adults will experience back pain.

2. A weak back is the most common cause of low back pain.　　True　　False

   Answer: False. The most common cause of low back pain is weak abdominal muscles.

3. Exercise can improve poor posture.　　True　　False

   Answer: True. Specific strength and flexibility exercises can help to realign the spine.

4. Asthmatics and arthritics should never participate in aerobic activity.　　True　　False

   Answer: False. With a physician's approval and with a few exercise modifications, aerobic activity can improve the overall health of people with asthma or arthritis.

Evaluating Your Health History

It is important that you complete a health history evaluation before beginning an aerobic dance program. There are a number of conditions that require a physician's approval before you exercise. Although few circumstances will prevent your participation in physical activity altogether, certain situations require special program modifications. Answer the following questions:

1. Do you have a history of any of the following conditions?

Heart problem	Yes	No
High blood pressure*	Yes	No
High cholesterol*	Yes	No
Respiratory problems	Yes	No
Diabetes	Yes	No
Surgery within the last 3 months	Yes	No
Major illness or hospitalization in the last 3 months	Yes	No
Major muscle, joint, or back disorder	Yes	No

2. Are you over 45 years of age? Yes No
3. Would you consider yourself to be obese? Yes No
4. Are you pregnant? Yes No
5. Are you taking any medication?† Yes No

---

* If you do not know your blood pressure or cholesterol level, it is wise to find out before you begin an exercise program.

† If you are currently taking medication, check with your physician to be sure that the medication will not interfere with your ability to exercise safely.

If you answered yes to any of the questions above, ask your physician whether it is safe for you to participate in an aerobic dance class. Be sure to follow your physician's advice and the exercise modifications listed in Table 2.1.

Testing Your Posture

Not only is poor posture unattractive, but it can also lead to serious injury. Spinal malalignment is the major cause of many common aches and pains suffered by adults. Eight out of ten adults will experience some form of pain in the lower part of the back. A smaller but significant number will be plagued by neck and shoulder discomfort.

Table 2.1　　**Exercise Modifications for Health Conditions**

Health Condition	Exercise Modifications
Arthritis	1. Begin physical activity with a long and gradual warm-up. 2. Emphasize stretching exercises. 3. Minimize high impacts on the feet. 4. Avoid the use of weights during aerobic activity. 5. Stop any exercise that causes undue pain in the joints.
Asthma	1. Begin physical activity with a long and gradual warm-up.
Back pain (especially in the lower back)	1. Avoid the use of weights during aerobic activity. 2. Avoid exercises that require bending and touching the floor or trunk-twisting movements. 3. Stop any activity that causes undue back pain.
Heart disease and high blood pressure	1. Avoid high exercise intensities during aerobic activity. 2. Avoid static strengthening exercises (isometric contractions). 3. Avoid exercising with your arms at or above shoulder level for an extended period of time. 4. Avoid lifting excessively heavy weights. 5. Never hold your breath when doing strength exercises.
Joint discomfort (such as runner's knee, tennis elbow)	1. Avoid those exercises and activities that place undue stress on the affected joint. 2. Stop any activity that causes excessive joint pain.
Obesity	1. Avoid high-impact activities. 2. Avoid the use of weights during aerobic exercise.

Continued

Table 2.1—Continued

Health Condition	Exercise Modifications
Pregnancy	1. Do not begin a vigorous exercise program at this time if you have not been exercising regularly.
	2. After the first trimester, minimize participating in high-impact activities.
	3. After the fourth month of pregnancy, avoid exercising while lying on your back.
	4. Avoid high exercise intensities during aerobic exercise.
	5. Avoid excessive stretching.

A healthy back has three natural curves, including a slight forward curve in the neck and lower back regions and a small backward curve in the upper back (see Figure 2.1). Good posture requires that you keep these curves in balanced alignment. When the spine is out of alignment, stress is placed on the discs between the vertebrae. Years of improperly loading the spine will eventually result in back, neck, or shoulder pain.

Tight muscles and opposing weak muscles tug and push the spine out of alignment. For example, weak abdominal muscles with corresponding tight hip and lower back muscles result in too much curvature of the lower back, whereas weak back muscles and tight muscles in the back of the thigh create too little curvature. Similarly, the curve of the upper back is exaggerated when the muscles of the upper back are weak and the chest muscles are tight.

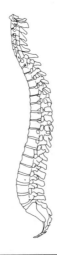

FIGURE 2.1
The natural curves of the
spine (side view).

Use Table 2.2 to identify specific postural deviations. Have a friend evaluate you from the side or have someone take a picture of you so that you can evaluate your own posture. Always assume a comfortable and normal stance when testing posture.

If you have good posture, you should be able to draw an imaginary line that passes straight through your ear, the front portion of your shoulder, the center of your hip, behind your kneecap, and in front of your ankle bone.

Table 2.2   Testing Your Posture

	Swayback Posture	Flat-back Posture	Good Posture
Chin	____ Tilted up or forward	____ Tilted down or pushed back	____ Centered
Shoulders	____ Rounded forward	____ Pushed too far back	____ Centered
Abdomen	____ Protruding	____ Flat	____ Flat
Lower back	____ Too much arch	____ Too flat	____ Slight arch
Knees	____ Hyper-extended	____ Too much knee bend	____ Straight

Many postural deviations can be corrected by consciously realigning your spine whenever you catch yourself standing or sitting incorrectly. Since a number of spinal malalignments are also associated with tight and weak muscles, a regular exercise program can improve posture. Table 2.3 provides exercise remedies for the most common postural deviations.

Testing Your Flexibility

Testing flexibility is very important because tight muscles can affect both appearance and performance and may be responsible for common joint aches and pains. It is always wise to test your flexibility and correct any problems that you might have before beginning a vigorous exercise program.

There is no single test to assess your flexibility, because flexibility is joint specific. This simply means that flexibility can vary tremendously from one joint to another. Therefore, you must check the flexibility of all your major joints and perform stretching exercises for each specific joint that requires improved flexibility.

Table 2.3   Posture Deviations and Remedies

| | Exercise Remedy* | |
Postural Flaw	Stretching	Strengthening
Rounded shoulders	Underarm press Overarm press	Elbow press
Protruding abdomen		Pelvic tilts Curl-ups Diagonal curls
Excessive arch of the lower back	Back curls Knees to chest Lunges	
Flat back	Reverse lunge Leg pull	
Hyperextended knees	Heel pull	

*   Refer to Chapters 4 and 5 for exercise descriptions.

To test your flexibility, use the following guidelines and follow the directions in Table 2.4.

1. Dress comfortably.
2. Find a partner to assist you or use a mirror.
3. Place yourself in the starting body position.
4. Slowly stretch as far as you can until the point of tension (you should not experience pain).
5. Do not bounce or force any positions.
6. Discontinue any test that causes undue pain and consult your instructor.
7. Compare your final position with the passing position.
8. If you are tight, perform the suggested exercise remedies regularly.

Testing Your Strength

To protect the integrity of your joints, the strength of muscles on both sides of a joint must be balanced. If the muscle on one side of a joint is significantly stronger than the muscle on the other side, this imbalance can produce changes in body alignment, which can ultimately lead to injury, especially as you become more active. Unfortunately, measuring the relative strength between opposing muscle groups often requires expensive and sophisticated equipment. There is, however, a simple test for measuring the relative strength between the hip flexors and the abdominals. This is particularly important because weakness in the abdominals as compared to the hip flexors can often lead to low back pain. Strong hip flexors tend to pull your lower spine into a swayback position if the abdominal muscles are weak. In contrast, strong abdominal muscles can help maintain a desirable curvature of the lumbar spine (the lower back region).

Abdominal Strength Test Precautions

1. Do not perform any of the abdominal tests if you currently suffer from low back pain or have recently had a back injury or back surgery.
2. Before taking the abdominal muscle balance test, take the abdominal curl-up test. If you do not pass the curl-up test, do not attempt the muscle balance test.
3. When performing the abdominal muscle balance test, be sure that your partner supports your legs as soon as your back pulls off the floor to minimize the stress on your lower back.

Table 2.4   Testing Flexibility

Body Part and Directions	Passing Description	Passing Position	Not Passing Position	Exercise Remedy*
SHOULDERS				
Reach over the shoulder to the opposite shoulder blade.	Touching the top of the opposite shoulder blade.			Elbow press Overarm shoulder press
Reach behind the lower back and up to the opposite shoulder blade.	Touching the bottom of the opposite shoulder blade.			Underarm shoulder press
LOWER BACK				
Lying on your back, pull both knees to the chest.	Both knees touch the chest.			Knees to chest Back curls
FRONT OF HIPS				
Lying on your back, pull one knee to the chest.	Extended leg remains straight and on the floor.			Lunges

Table 2.4 Continued

Body Part and Directions	Passing Description	Passing Position	Not Passing Position	Exercise Remedy*
BACK OF THIGHS Lying on your back, extend one leg up as far as possible, keeping both legs straight.	Both legs remain straight and the leg in the air is perpendicular to the floor.			Reverse lunge Leg pull
FRONT OF THIGHS† Lying on your stomach, pull the foot toward the buttocks, keeping the head and shoulders down and the legs together.	Heel comfortably touches the buttocks.			Heel pull
CALF Standing with the heels, buttocks, shoulders, and head against a wall, raise one forefoot off the floor, keeping both knees straight (not hyper-extended) and the heels down.	Ball of the foot should clear the floor by at least two finger widths.		Less than two finger widths under the ball of the foot	Toe raises Heel press Toe pull

* See Chapter 4 for specific exercise descriptions.

† Do not perform this test if you experience knee pain or if you just recently had knee surgery.

Abdominal Curl-Up Test

Starting position: Lie on your back with your knees bent and your feet flat on the floor (Figure 2.2).

Test: Place your hands behind your head, elbows pointing to the sides. Without pulling your head with your hands, slowly lift the head and shoulders off the floor, keeping your lower back down (Figure 2.3). Hold for ten slow counts, then slowly lower your shoulders and head down to the floor. If you were able to hold the raised position comfortably, you have passed the curl-up test and may proceed to the abdominal muscle balance test.

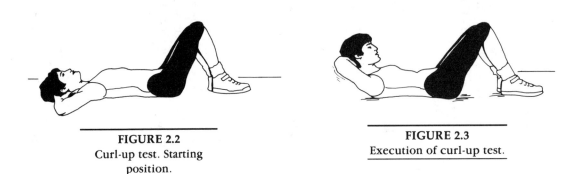

FIGURE 2.2
Curl-up test. Starting
position.

FIGURE 2.3
Execution of curl-up test.

Abdominal Muscle Balance Test

Your abdominal muscles should be strong enough to lower your legs to the floor. If they are not, your lower back will pull up off the floor before your legs reach a horizontal position. A raised lower back indicates that the psoas muscles (hip flexors) have taken over the task of lowering the legs. The farther you can lower your legs with the abdominals and not the hip flexors, the better the muscular balance is between these two muscle groups.

To perform the test, find a partner to assist you. Lie on the floor with your arms above the head and both legs perpendicular to the floor. This position should force your lower back to be flat against the floor. Have your partner kneel down beside you, placing one hand on the floor by the small of your back and the other hand a few inches away from your legs (Figure 2.4).

Slowly lower both legs to the floor. As soon as your partner feels your lower back lift off the floor, he or she will support your legs while determining the angle of your legs to the floor. Your partner will then assist you in bending your knees and pulling your legs toward your chest.

Test Results: (shown in Figure 2.5)

Passing—legs are 30 degrees or less from the floor.
Not passing—legs are more than 30 degrees from the floor.

To improve abdominal strength, regularly perform pelvic tilts, curl-ups, and diagonal curls (see Chapter 5 for exercise descriptions).

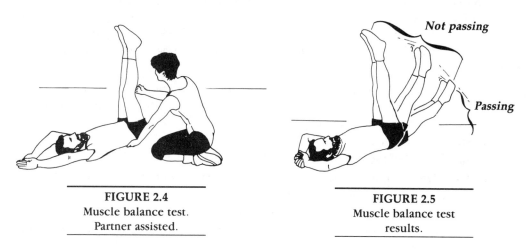

FIGURE 2.4
Muscle balance test.
Partner assisted.

FIGURE 2.5
Muscle balance test
results.

Testing Your Aerobic Fitness

To help you determine the appropriate exercise progression during your aerobic dance class, you must first know your present level of aerobic fitness. If you progress too quickly by exercising too hard, too often, or too long, you greatly increase your risk of becoming injured.

Refer to Table 2.5 to estimate your present level of aerobic fitness based on the intensity, duration, and frequency of your normal weekly physical activity.

Table 2.5   Estimated Aerobic Fitness Level

Physical Activity	Poor	Fair	Good
Times per week (frequency)	0–1	2	3 or more
Length of continuous activity (duration)	Less than 10 minutes	11–19 minutes	20 or more minutes
Vigor of activity (intensity)	Normal breathing	Moderate breathing	Deep breathing

If you do not presently exercise at least three times per week for twenty or more continuous minutes at an intensity that causes your breathing to be deep and sustained, you need to begin your aerobic activity slowly. Start with ten minutes of aerobic dance per session until you are comfortable with the workload. As the aerobic activity becomes easier, add five minutes per session until you reach at least twenty consecutive minutes.

A step test will allow you to measure improvements in your aerobic fitness over time. The faster your heart rate recovers back toward resting levels after a fixed amount of exercise, the better your aerobic fitness. To take the step test, find a step measuring anywhere from eight to twelve inches. Use a metronome or a prerecorded audiotape to keep a consistent and audible beat. Make sure that you are well rested before taking the test. Follow these instructions:

1. Step up with the left foot, up with the right foot, down with the left foot, and down with the right foot (Figure 2.6) to a cadence of 96 steps per minute (use a metronome or an audiotape).
2. Step for three minutes.
3. Sit down after three minutes and find your pulse.
4. After five seconds, count your pulse for fifteen seconds and multiply by four.
5. Record your recovery heart rate.
6. Retest each month, looking for a decrease in recovery heart rate. For comparative purposes, be sure to use a step of the same height each time you test your aerobic fitness.

If your step test recovery heart rate significantly decreases from one test to another, your aerobic fitness is improving.

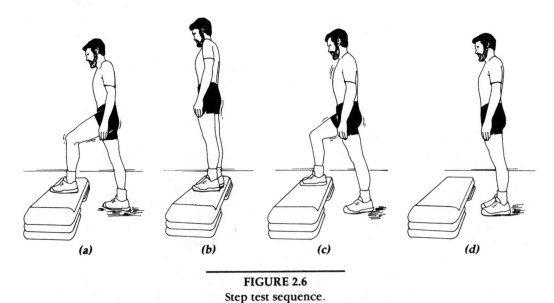

(a) *(b)* *(c)* *(d)*

FIGURE 2.6
Step test sequence.

KEY POINTS IN CHAPTER 2

1. Complete a health history evaluation before starting an aerobic dance program. If you suffer from any of the conditions indicated on the evaluation form in Table 2.1, consult your physician before participating in an aerobic dance class. Once you begin your program, be sure to make appropriate exercise modifications.

2. Poor posture can increase your risk of injury during exercise. Spinal malalignment is the major cause for back, neck, and shoulder pain. Before starting an aerobic dance program, test for postural deficiencies and correct any obvious problems.

3. Poor flexibility can affect your performance in an aerobic dance class. Test the tightness of each of your major muscles and stretch those that are tight.

4. To avoid injury, it is important to maintain a balance between the strength of muscles on both sides of a joint. Of particular concern is the lower back region, because most adults experience some form of back pain. Test the strength of your abdominal muscles. If you discover a weakness, be sure to strengthen these muscles.

5. Progressing too quickly in your aerobic dance class can increase your risk of becoming injured. Determine your present level of aerobic fitness and progress accordingly.

3 Getting Started in an Aerobic Dance Program

TEST YOUR KNOWLEDGE

Answer true or false to the following statements:

1. Aerobic dance can help to strengthen your bones.   True   False

   Answer: True. Activities such as aerobic dance that involve an impact between the feet and the floor increase the strength of bones which reduces the likelihood of developing osteoporosis (loss of bone density).

2. When testing a shoe for flexibility, the shoe should bend in the middle as you curl the toe and heel together.   True   False

   Answer: False. The shoe should always bend under the ball of the foot, which is where your foot naturally bends when you walk, run, or jump.

3. Aerobic dancing on a thick mat is ideal because it significantly improves shock absorption.   True   False

   Answer: False. Although it is true that a thick mat does improve shock absorption, it also reduces stability, which could result in ankle sprains and falls.

4. Clothing with a high percentage of nylon is appropriate for aerobic dance because it helps to keep you cool.   True   False

   Answer: False. Cotton fabrics are ideal for aerobic dance because unlike nylon, they absorb perspiration and allow for optimal evaporation.

What Is Aerobic Dance?

The term *aerobic dance* was coined by Jackie Sorensen in the late 1960s. Developed as a way of improving aerobic fitness by means of dancing continuously and vigorously to popular music in a group setting, aerobic dance became one of the fastest-growing leisure activities. This dynamic and exciting exercise program has attracted more than 24 million participants in the United States alone. Exercise enthusiasts can choose among many forms of aerobic dance, ranging from calisthenics and jazz to cardiofunk and water aerobics. Participants can also select specific class formats that range from low-, moderate-, or high-impact aerobics to continuous, interval, or circuit training.

Benefits of Aerobic Dance

The health benefits associated with regular participation in aerobic dance (some of which have been mentioned previously) include the following:

1. Reduced risk of developing heart disease
2. Being able to perform more work with less fatigue
3. Recovering from fatigue more quickly
4. Reduced risk of developing osteoporosis (loss of bone density)
5. Being able to perform daily tasks with greater ease
6. Reduced risk of developing common aches and pains such as back, neck, and shoulder discomfort
7. Improved physical appearance (less fat and greater muscle definition)
8. Improved posture and body mechanics
9. Improved athletic performance
10. Reduced levels of stress

Choosing an Aerobic Dance Class

When selecting an aerobic dance program, be sure that the instructor is well qualified. In addition, look for an instructor whose style of aerobic dance is to your personal liking. Use the checklist in Table 3.1 when choosing an aerobic dance program.

Table 3.1 Checklist for Selecting an Aerobic Dance Program

		Yes	No
1.	Instructor is certified or has a degree in a fitness-related field.	___	___
2.	Some form of fitness assessment is administered.	___	___
3.	Shoes are required.	___	___
4.	Instructor is visible to everyone in the room.	___	___
5.	Instructor can be heard by everyone in the room.	___	___
6.	There is enough space for everyone to move comfortably.	___	___
7.	The program addresses the five components of health-related fitness.*	___	___
8.	The instructor uses safe and effective exercise techniques.†	___	___
9.	The instructor periodically wanders around the room, observing and correcting technique when necessary.	___	___
10.	The instructor shows genuine concern for class participants.	___	___

* Components of health-related fitness are discussed in Chapter 1.

† Safe and effective exercise techniques are discussed in Chapters 4 through 7.

The more questions to which you answered yes in Table 3.1, the safer and more effective the aerobic dance program.

Components of an Aerobic Dance Class

A sound aerobic dance class includes activities that address the five components of health-related fitness: cardiovascular endurance, muscular strength and endurance, flexibility, and body composition. Table 3.2 summarizes the component parts of an aerobic dance program.

Table 3.2   Components of an Aerobic Dance Program

Activity	Duration (minutes)	Purpose	Type of Movements
Warm-up and pre-stretch	10–15	Prepares the body for aerobic exercise; enhances flexibility	Rhythmic movements of the large muscles of the body; specific static stretches held for at least 10 seconds
Aerobic dance	20–30	Improves cardiovascular endurance and body composition	Continuous, vigorous, and rhythmic exercise of the large muscles of the body
Aerobic cool down	3–5	Allows the body to gradually recover to a normal level of activity	Slower rhythmic movements of the large muscles of the body
Isolation work (floor work)	10–20	Enhances strength and muscular endurance	Repetitive contractions of specific muscles using some form of resistance
Final stretch	5–15	Elongates muscles that have been contracting during the aerobic dance segment; enhances overall flexibility	Static stretching exercises held for 10–30 seconds

Sticking with Your Aerobic Dance Program

Sticking with your exercise program is not always easy. People often quit exercising because their program fails to meet their personal needs or expectations. Fortunately, there are a number of factors that can increase the likelihood of long-term participation in an aerobic dance program.

Fitness Assessment and Periodic Re-evaluation: Knowing your current level of fitness will ensure that you are exercising at an appropriate level. In addition, periodic re-evaluation will help you determine the extent of improvement and success that you have achieved with your exercise program.

Goal Setting: People with clear, specific, and realistic exercise goals are more likely to feel successful with their fitness programs and are thus more inclined to commit to exercise over a longer period of time.

Record Keeping of Progress: The most effective way to determine improvements in fitness is to monitor your progress by keeping careful records of your exercise activities. Visible improvements in fitness often lead to greater motivation and exercise compliance.

Progression at a Slow Rate: The key to long-term participation in exercise is to stay injury free. Do not be in a hurry. The best way to minimize musculoskeletal injuries is to progress gradually.

Program Variety and Fun: You are more likely to stay motivated if your program is exciting. Look for an aerobic dance class that is stimulating and offers plenty of program variety and fun.

Setting Exercise Goals

Without a specific idea of what you want to accomplish from an aerobic dance program, your exercise efforts are likely to be haphazard and wasteful. Goal setting will help you design an exercise program that is right for your needs, and it will also help you commit to exercise over a longer period of time. One of the most effective ways to set exercise goals is to use the SMART technique. This method will ensure that your exercise goals are Specific, Measurable, Action-oriented, Realistic, and Timed.

Specific: You must decide what you would specifically like to accomplish from your aerobic dance program. For example, you may want to lose weight, improve muscle definition, or reduce the risk of developing coronary heart disease. Write down your specific expectations.

Measurable: Unless a goal is measurable, you have no way of knowing whether it has been accomplished. Fortunately, most specific exercise goals can be measured. For example, you can assess changes in your flexibility, aerobic fitness, strength, and even sports performance. In order to measure your exercise improvement, however, you must first determine your present level of fitness and health.

Action-oriented: The most effective means for accomplishing your exercise goals is to develop a written plan. This plan must be detailed and realistic. Each chosen exercise should serve a specific purpose to meet your personal needs. The plan should include both short-term and long-term goals. Short-term goals will give you a sense of immediate accomplishment and a feeling of success from day to day or week to week. Long-term goals will focus on the desired final outcome. For example, losing sixty pounds is a long-term goal, whereas losing two pounds per week is a short-term goal.

Your written plan should be reviewed periodically to ensure that your exercise program is indeed accomplishing your desired goals. If your action plan appears unrealistic, change it. Be aware, however, that it takes six to eight weeks to change an old behavior pattern. Try to determine whether your discomfort with the program is because of the newness of the activity or because your expectations are unrealistic.

Realistic: People often quit exercising because they are disillusioned when their exercise program fails to accomplish the anticipated results. In many cases, the exercise goals were unrealistic from the start. When setting exercise goals, you must be realistic about your genetic potential. If you are extremely muscular and large boned, you will never look like a high-fashion model, no matter how much you exercise. Similarly, if you have very long limbs and a small musculoskeletal frame, you are not likely to look like a body builder.

When setting realistic goals, your exercise preferences must be taken into account. Select activities that you enjoy doing and make sure that your exercise program fits conveniently into your current life-style. If you schedule aerobic dance at a time when you have to rush to class, leaving little time for travel, taking a shower, or changing your workout clothes, your attendance is likely to suffer. Finally, it will be much easier to exercise regularly if you select an aerobic dance class facility that is conveniently located near your school, work, or home.

Timed: Without a target date, you are not fully committed to your exercise goals. A timed goal provides powerful motivation for long-term participation in an exercise program. Make sure that the time required to complete the goal is realistic. Losing ten pounds of fat in one week is impossible. A more realistic goal would be to lose one to two pounds per week.

The following is an example of a SMART exercise goal:

To improve my cardiovascular endurance, I will participate in an aerobic dance program three times per week (Specific and Realistic). I will improve my step test score from a recovery heart rate of 122 beats per minute to 100 beats per minute over a period of six months (Realistic, Measurable, and Timed). I will begin my program with a slow progression of ten minutes of aerobic activity, adding five minutes every week until I can comfortably participate in thirty consecutive minutes of aerobic exercise (Action-oriented). My long-term goal is to reduce my recovery heart rate by 22 beats per minute in a six-month period. My short-term goal is to decrease my recovery heart rate by about 4 beats per minute each month.

Choosing Aerobic Dance Shoes

The most important item of aerobic dance equipment that you will buy is a good pair of shoes. Essentially, shoes are an injury-prevention device that cushions and stabilizes your foot during movement. When buying a pair of shoes, you must consider your foot type and the type of floor on which you will be exercising. A shoe must provide a number of important features, including the following:

Comfort and Fit: Be sure that the shoes are not too wide (which causes too much movement of the foot inside the shoe) or too tight (which creates too much pressure on certain portions of the foot). The arch of your foot should be comfortably supported while your heel fits snugly into the shoe. Make sure that your toes have enough room for some movement.

Cushioning: The shoe should have adequate cushioning under the ball of the foot and the heel. Jump up and down in the shoes to test for shock absorption. If the shoes do not cushion your feet as you land from a jump, they may not provide enough shock absorption.

Stability: Your foot should remain firmly in place inside the shoe. During lateral movement, your foot should not roll excessively from side to side.

Flexibility: Because your foot bends near the ball of the foot, be sure that the shoe bends under the forefoot portion, not under the arch of the foot. A good test for flexibility is to bend the shoe while holding it in your hands. If the shoe bends in the center, it is poorly designed. If the shoe does not bend at all, it is too stiff and you will experience discomfort during exercise.

Traction: Your shoes should move smoothly across the exercise surface. If they stick or slide too much, you are more likely to trip or fall during class.

Certain individuals have unique shoe requirements. If you have any of the conditions shown in Table 3.3, make sure that your shoes provide you with the special characteristics listed.

What You Should Know about Floors

Even with an excellent pair of shoes, you may experience discomfort and eventual injury if the surface on which you are exercising is poor. As with your shoes, a floor must provide the following characteristics: (1) adequate shock absorption to cushion vertical impact forces; (2) stability to control lateral movements; (3) traction to allow the foot to move smoothly across the surface; and (4) resiliency to allow the surface to spring back to its original shape.

Table 3.3   Shoe Characteristics for Various Health Conditions

Condition	Shoe Characteristics
Shin splints	Good stability and cushioning
Knee pain	Stability
Ankle sprains	Lateral stability
Flat feet	Stability
High arch	Good cushioning and arch support

Floor surfaces can be covered either with carpet, wood, or vinyl. The section of the floor directly below the top surface is usually made of foam padding, springs or wood boards. The ideal surface provides an adequate balance among shock absorption, stability, traction, and resiliency. Keep in mind that too much cushioning, such as that found in thick mats, will provide good shock absorption but poor stability. Your foot will sink deeply into the soft mat, making it difficult to move safely from side to side. Floor surfaces that provide too much traction, such as a thick carpet, can cause ankle sprains, tripping, and falling. A floor that is too rigid, such as concrete, will provide great stability but poor shock absorption, resulting in injuries such as shin and lower back pain. An excellent aerobic dance surface is a hard wood sprung floor.

Selecting Aerobic Dance Clothing

During vigorous activity, your body produces a great deal of heat. To maintain core or inner body temperature, your body perspires as a way of removing excess internal heat. It is very important not to interfere with the cooling process. Selecting proper clothing can enhance temperature regulation.

By minimizing the amount of skin that is covered, you allow heat to dissipate more efficiently. Today's aerobic dance fashions include bike shorts, three-quarter-length tights, sleeveless leotards, short tops, and t-shirts, all of which effectively expose your skin to the surrounding air.

The best fabrics for aerobic dance clothing are made with cotton. Cotton materials are cooler because they absorb sweat and allow for optimal evaporation. Many aerobic dance clothes use fabrics that are either 100 percent cotton or a blend containing some percentage of cotton.

Never wear an impermeable garment such as a rubber warm-up suit. This practice impairs heat loss and could lead to serious injuries such as heat exhaustion and heat stroke.

When choosing your aerobic dance clothing, select styles that are comfortable. Avoid zippers and belts with large buckles, as they may constrict movement.

KEY POINTS IN CHAPTER 3

1. More than 24 million people participate in aerobic dance in the United States.

2. Participants can select from many class formats, such as high-, moderate-, and low-impact aerobics and circuit or interval training. Styles of aerobic dance vary from cardiofunk and jazz to simple calisthenic movements.

3. There are many health benefits associated with regular participation in aerobic dance.

4. When selecting an aerobic dance program, find an instructor who is well qualified and who uses safe and effective exercise techniques.

5. A sound aerobic dance class includes ten to fifteen minutes of a warm-up and pre-stretch, twenty to thirty minutes of aerobic dance, three to five minutes of a cool-down, ten to twenty minutes of isolation work, and five to fifteen minutes of postaerobic stretching.

6. For long-term participation in an aerobic dance program, assess and periodically re-evaluate your current level of physical fitness, set exercise goals, keep records of your progress, find a program that offers variety and fun, and always progress slowly.

7. Set exercise goals and be sure that they are specific, measurable, action-oriented, realistic, and timed (SMART).

8. Select an aerobic dance shoe that fits your foot comfortably and provides adequate cushioning, stability, flexibility, and traction.

9. Perform aerobic dance on a surface that provides adequate shock absorption, stability, traction, and resiliency.

10. Wear exercise clothing that absorbs perspiration, allows heat to dissipate effectively, and does not restrict movement.

4 *Flexibility and Stretching*

TEST YOUR KNOWLEDGE

Answer true or false to the following statements:

1. Stretching exercises can help to firm and tone muscle. 　　　　　　　　　　　　　　True　　False

   Answer: False. Stretching exercises elongate tight muscles.

2. Stretching exercises can alleviate common aches and pains such as back and neck discomfort. 　　True　　False

   Answer: True. Stretching exercises can elongate tight muscles that tend to pull the spine out of alignment, thus causing various aches and pains.

3. The best stretching technique is ballistic stretching, which involves bouncing or pulsing movements. 　True　　False

   Answer: False. Although ballistic stretching will elongate the muscle, it can also result in overstretching and possibly in tearing the muscle. In addition, ballistic stretching often leads to greater postexercise soreness.

4. Standing toe touches are an excellent exercise for stretching the lower back and the back of the thighs. 　True　　False

   Answer: False. Although this exercise will stretch the lower back and the back of the thighs, bending forward from the waist while standing places uneven compression on the discs of the lower spine and could result in a back injury.

Principles and Importance of Flexibility

Flexibility describes the range of possible motion at each of your joints. Poor flexibility in some of your joints may be due to excessive fat, scar tissue, or tight ligaments and tendons surrounding the joint. It is more likely, however, that your inflexibility is caused by tight muscles. Fortunately, tight muscles can be elongated using various stretching techniques.

Although flexibility exercises will not firm your muscles or remove fat from a body part, they can affect your personal appearance. The way in which you hold your body (your posture) is partially a result of the tightness of your muscles. For example, if you have tight chest muscles you probably also have rounded shoulders. Similarly, if you have tight lower back and hip muscles, you are likely to have a swayback posture. Most postural deviations are unattractive. Rounded shoulders make you look stocky by appearing to reduce your height; a swayback posture causes your abdomen to protrude, giving the illusion of a thick waistline. Regular stretching can improve your posture and can therefore enhance your appearance.

Adequate levels of flexibility can also improve your exercise performance. Increased range of motion in the joints allows you to bend, reach, jump, and stride farther. Lack of flexibility can cause poor body mechanics, which in turn result in improper, awkward, or uncoordinated movements.

Finally, adequate flexibility helps you to maintain the spine in proper alignment. Tight muscles, in contrast, pull the spine and other joints into mechanically inefficient positions, causing aggravating pain. The most common complaints involve discomfort in the back, neck, and shoulders. Unfortunately, the discomfort becomes more pronounced when levels of physical activity are increased because greater stress is placed on these sensitive areas. A regular stretching program can help prevent many of the common aches and pains that occur in adulthood.

Myths about Flexibility

1. **Myth:** Stretching exercises such as trunk twisting or side bends will firm the area being exercised.

   Fact: Stretching exercises simply elongate muscles. To become firmer and stronger, muscles must contract against some form of resistance.

2. **Myth:** Stretching exercises such as toe touching will remove fat from the area being exercised.

   Fact: The greater the energy expenditure required from an activity, the more calories are burned and the more fat is removed from all the fat stores in your body. Stretching exercises require very little energy expenditure.

3. **Myth:** If you are flexible in one or two joints, you are flexible in all of your joints.

   Fact: Flexibility is joint specific. This means that you may be very flexible in one joint and not at all flexible in another joint.

Stretching Technique and Guidelines

To improve your flexibility, you want to safely and effectively elongate your muscles. Holding an exercise position, called *static stretching,* is generally safer than bouncing or ballistic stretching. When you bounce vigorously, there is always a danger that you will overstretch and possibly tear a muscle. In addition, research has shown that muscle soreness is greater following ballistic stretching than after static stretching. Always stretch to the point of tension in the muscle, not pain. Pain is the body's way of telling you that something is not right. If you are in pain, you have gone too far.

You should always warm up for about three to five minutes before stretching. A warm-up helps your body prepare for flexibility exercises by increasing the muscle temperature, which in turn improves the elasticity of the muscles. Although you do not want to be out of breath, you should experience a slightly higher heart rate and feel a little warmer following the warm-up exercises. To warm up, perform large, rhythmic movements of the body such as marches, step touches, and step points along with shoulder, elbow, and arm circles.

Stretching for five to ten minutes before your aerobic exercise will help to prepare your body for vigorous exercise. Increasing your flexibility will enhance your aerobic dance performance and may reduce your risk of injury. Stretching for five to fifteen minutes after vigorous activity will elongate the muscles that have been contracting through a limited range of motion during exercise and will also improve your overall flexibility. You will probably find it easier to stretch after vigorous exercise because your muscles will be warm and your joints well lubricated. For this reason, you may want to hold your stretches for at least thirty seconds following aerobic exercise.

The following guidelines will help you to perform stretching exercises safely and effectively.

1. Wear clothing that will not constrict your movements.
2. Warm up for about three to five minutes before stretching.
3. Move slowly into each position and hold for at least ten seconds.
4. Breathe normally; do not hold your breath.
5. Stretch both sides of the body.
6. Stretch until you feel mild tension in the muscle. Never stretch to the point of pain.
7. Find the exercise position that is most comfortable for you. If a particular stretch is uncomfortable, choose an alternative exercise position that stretches the same muscles.

8. Relax as much as possible when you are stretching. Tightening the muscles that you are trying to stretch is counterproductive.

9. Stretch all the major muscles that will be used during your aerobic dance routines. Increased joint range of motion will greatly enhance your comfort and aerobic dance performance.

10. Stretch after aerobic exercise. Attempt to hold each stretch for at least thirty seconds.

11. Avoid hazardous exercise positions (see the section ''Risky Stretching Exercises'').

12. Do not continue to exercise if any position causes unusual discomfort. Seek the advice of your instructor or physician.

Stretching Exercises before Aerobic Activity

The following stretching exercises will help to prepare your body for aerobic exercise. A sample warm-up routine follows the description of the exercises.

Body Part: Neck

EXERCISE: Head tilts [Figure 4.1 (a) through (d)].

Starting Position: Standing.

Movement: Slowly lower the right ear toward the right shoulder. Repeat to the left side.

Tip: Do not lift the shoulders.

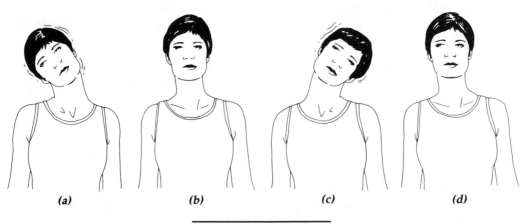

(a)   (b)   (c)   (d)

FIGURE 4.1
Head tilt sequence.

EXERCISE: Head rotations [Figure 4.2 (a) through (d)].

Starting Position: Standing.

Movement: Turn the head to the right and look over the right shoulder. Repeat to the left side.

Tip: Do not rotate the shoulders.

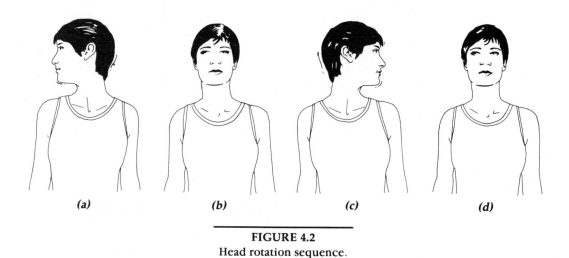

(a)   (b)   (c)   (d)

FIGURE 4.2
Head rotation sequence.

Body Part: Shoulders and Chest

EXERCISE: Overarm press (Figure 4.3).

Starting Position: Standing. Grip both hands above the head, bending the elbows slightly.

Movement: Gently press the arms backward.

Tips: Do not lock the elbows or arch the back. Both of these techniques place stress on the joints.

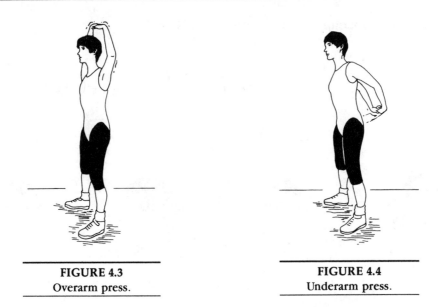

FIGURE 4.3
Overarm press.

FIGURE 4.4
Underarm press.

EXERCISE: Underarm press (Figure 4.4).

Starting Position: Standing. Grip both hands behind the back, bending the elbows slightly.

Movement: Gently press the arms upward.

Tips: Do not lock the elbows or bend forward at the waist. Both of these techniques place stress on the joints.

Body Part: Shoulders and Upper Arm

EXERCISE: Diagonal arm pull (Figure 4.5).

Starting Position: Standing. Place the right arm diagonally across the chest. Place the left hand on the right upper arm.

Movement: Gently pull the right arm across the body. Repeat on the left side.

Tip: If you experience pain in the shoulder joint, release some of the tension.

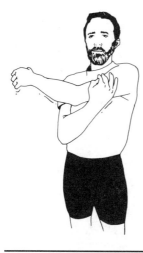

FIGURE 4.5
Diagonal arm pull.

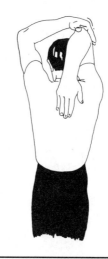

FIGURE 4.6
Elbow press.

EXERCISE: Elbow press (Figure 4.6).

Starting Position: Standing. Place the right hand behind the head and across to the left shoulder blade. Place the left hand on the right elbow.

Movement: Gently press the elbow downward with the left hand. Repeat on the left side.

Tip: Bend the head slightly forward for greater comfort. If you experience pain in the shoulder joint, release some of the tension.

Body Part: Waist

EXERCISE: Side bends (Figure 4.7).

Starting Position: Standing with the feet a little wider than shoulder-width apart, place the left hand on the left thigh for support. Extend the right arm upward diagonally.

Movement: Gently press the right arm toward the left side. Repeat on the left side.

Tip: Always support your weight on your thighs to minimize stress on the spine.

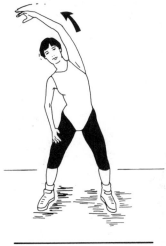

FIGURE 4.7
Side bends.

Body Part: Lower Back

EXERCISE: Supported back curls [Figure 4.8 (a) and (b)].

Starting Position: Standing. Bend the knees and lean over from the waist, placing the palms of the hands on the thighs.

Movement: Curl the back upward and hold.

Tips: Always support your weight on your upper thighs to avoid stress on the lower back. Do not lock the elbow joints.

EXERCISE: Unsupported back curls [Figure 4.9 (a) and (b)].

Starting Position: Standing. Turn the palms outward and grasp the hands in front of the chest.

Movement: Slowly drop the head and press the hands forward until the upper and lower back are curved.

Tips: Do not lock the knees or the elbows. Keep the shoulders down.

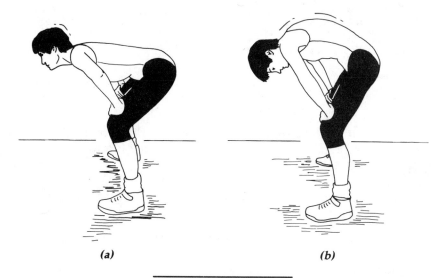

(a)   (b)

FIGURE 4.8
Supported back curls.
(*a*) Starting position.
(*b*) Movement.

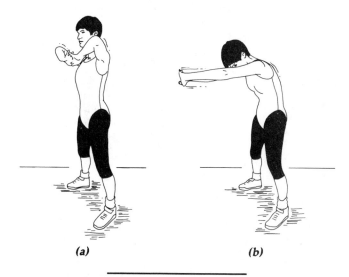

(a)   (b)

FIGURE 4.9
Unsupported back curls.
(*a*) Starting position.
(*b*) Movement.

Body Part: Front of Hips

EXERCISE: Standing lunge (Figure 4.10).

Starting Position: Standing. Place the right foot about twelve to eighteen inches in front of the left foot.

Movement: Tuck your buttocks tightly under your hips while contracting your abdominal muscles. You should feel the stretch in the front of the hip region of the rear leg. Repeat on the left side.

Tip: Do not lean backwards from the hips, as this places stress on the lower back.

EXERCISE: Kneeling lunge (Figure 4.11).

Starting Position: Extend the right leg to the rear, placing the right knee on the floor. Bend the left knee, making sure that it is directly over the left heel. Support your weight with both hands on the floor (one hand on each side of the left knee).

Movement: Tuck your buttocks tightly under your hips while contracting your abdominal muscles. You should feel the stretch in the front of the hip of the rear leg. Repeat on the left side.

Tips: Do not arch your back. Do not push the front knee over the toes, as this places excessive stress on the knee joint. Keep the rear knee on the floor to avoid overstretching the hip flexors.

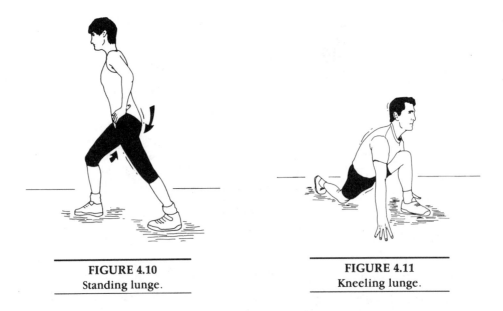

| **FIGURE 4.10** | **FIGURE 4.11** |
| Standing lunge. | Kneeling lunge. |

Body Part: Front of the Thigh

EXERCISE: Heel pull (Figure 4.12).

Starting Position: Stand and hold the right foot with the right hand, keeping the right knee pointing straight down.

Movement: Pull the right foot toward the buttocks. For greater stretch, tuck the buttocks tightly under the hips. Repeat on the left side.

Tips: Do not arch the back and do not pull your knee upward behind the back. Keep the knee pointing straight down. Discontinue this exercise if it hurts your knee.

Body Part: Back of the Thighs

EXERCISE: Reverse lunge (Figure 4.13).

Starting Position: Stand with the right leg fully extended in front of the left leg, which is bent. Lean forward, supporting your upper body weight on the top portion of your left thigh.

Movement: Slowly drop your weight downward until you feel mild tension in the back of the right thigh. Repeat on the left side.

Tips: Always support your body weight on your upper thigh. Do not lock the extended knee. Keep your hips facing forward.

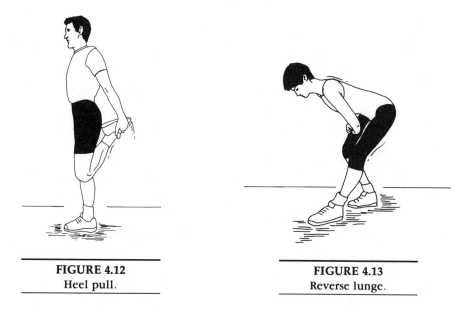

FIGURE 4.12
Heel pull.

FIGURE 4.13
Reverse lunge.

Body Part: Calf

EXERCISE: Toe raises (Figure 4.14).

Starting Position: Stand with the right leg extended in front of the left leg, which is bent. Bend forward, supporting your upper body weight on the top portion of your left thigh.

Movement: Raise the toes of the right foot, keeping the heel on the floor. Repeat on the left side.

Tips: Always support your body weight on your upper thigh. Do not lock the extended knee. Keep your hips facing forward.

EXERCISE: Heel press (Figure 4.15).

Starting Position: Standing. Place the left foot several feet in front of the right foot.

Movement: Press the right heel into the floor as you lean forward over the left leg. Repeat on the left side.

Tip: Keep the toes of the rear foot facing forward (not inward or outward).

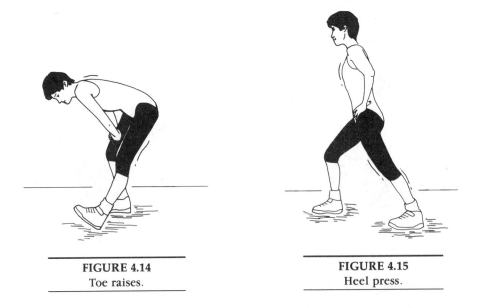

FIGURE 4.14
Toe raises.

FIGURE 4.15
Heel press.

Sample Warm-Up and Pre-Stretch Routine

Sequence	Counts	Direction	Step Pattern/Stretch*	Arm Movement*
1	16	In place	March	No arms
2	8	In place	March	4 overhead presses
3	8	In place	March	4 side presses
4	8	In place	March	4 press downs
5	8	In place	March	4 chest presses
6	4	In place	March	2 overhead presses
7	4	In place	March	2 side presses
8	4	In place	March	2 press downs
9	4	In place	March	2 chest presses
10	2	In place	March	1 overhead press
11	2	In place	March	1 side press
12	2	In place	March	1 press down
13	2	In place	March	1 chest press
14	8	Forward	March	Repeat arms for sequence 10–13
15	8	Backward	March	Repeat arms for sequence 10–13

Repeat sequence 14 and 15

16	8	In place	Step touch	No arms
17	8	In place	Step touch	4 alternating shoulder circles
18	8	In place	Step touch	4 alternating elbow circles
19	8	In place	Step touch	4 alternating arm circles

Repeat sequence 16–19

20	4	In place	Step touch	No arms
21	4	In place	Step touch	2 alternating shoulder circles
22	4	In place	Step touch	2 alternating elbow circles
23	4	In place	Step touch	2 alternating arm circles

Repeat sequence 20–23

24	8	In place	Step point	No arms
25	32	In place	Step point	16 arm swings
26	12	In place	Supported back curl	Hands on thighs
27	4	In place	Curl up to standing position	Arms at side of body
28	8	In place	Head tilts to right, then left	Arms at side of body

Repeat sequence 28 to the right

29	8	In place	Head rotations to the right, then left	Arms at side of body

Repeat sequence 29 to the left

30	16	In place	Overarm press	Arms above head
31	16	In place	Underarm press	Arms behind back
32	16	In place	Standing lunge (left hip)	8 chest presses
33	16	In place	Reverse lunge (right leg)	8 arm curls with left arm, right hand on left thigh
34	16	In place	Toe raises (right foot)	8 press downs with left arm, right hand on left thigh
35	16	In place	Heel pull (left leg)	Right arm overhead

Repeat sequence 32–35, stretching the other side of the body

36	8	In place	Step point	No arms
37	8	In place	Step heel	No arms
38	8	In place	Step point	4 L positions
39	8	In place	Step heel	4 press downs
40	8	Forward	Step point	4 L positions
41	8	Backward	Step heel	4 press downs

Repeat sequence 40 and 41 three more times

42	32	In place	March or jog	16 claps

---

* See Chapter 7 for a description of the step patterns and arm movements.

Stretching Exercises after Aerobic Activity

The following exercises are performed in a seated or reclined position, allowing you to relax into your final stretches. For greater variety and a more complete stretch after aerobic exercise, incorporate the stretches for the neck, shoulder, and chest (pp. 30–33) while in a seated position. A sample poststretch routine follows the exercises.

Body Part: Lower Back

EXERCISE: Knees to chest (Figure 4.16).

Starting Position: Lie on your back.

Movement: Gently pull both knees to your chest.

Tip: To reduce stress on the knee joints, grasp behind the thighs rather than around the knees.

Body Part: Back of Thighs

EXERCISE: Leg pull (Figure 4.17).

Starting Position: Lie on your back, knees bent, feet flat on floor.

Movement: Gently pull the right leg toward your chest. Keep your head and shoulders down. Repeat on the left side.

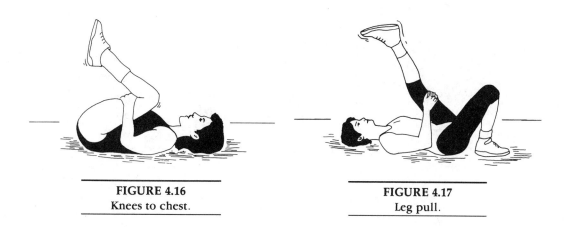

FIGURE 4.16
Knees to chest.

FIGURE 4.17
Leg pull.

Tips: To reduce stress on the knee joint, grasp behind the thigh rather than behind the knee or the calf.

If you cannot reach your leg without taking your head and shoulders off the floor, place a towel around your thigh and gently pull on the towel (Figure 4.18).

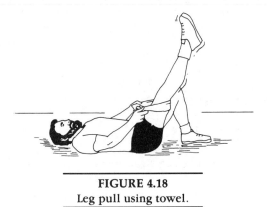

FIGURE 4.18
Leg pull using towel.

Body Part: Inner Thigh

EXERCISE: Straddle (Figure 4.19).

Starting Position: Lie on your back and pull both knees to your chest. Separate your knees, placing your hands on the inside of your knees.

Movement: Gently press the knees outward and downward.

Tip: If you are flexible in the hip joint, you may want to fully extend the legs from the knees (Figure 4.20).

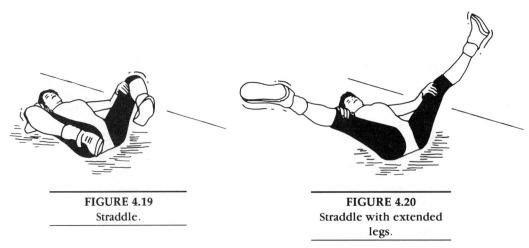

FIGURE 4.19
Straddle.

FIGURE 4.20
Straddle with extended legs.

Body Part: Outer Thigh

EXERCISE: Crossed leg press (Figure 4.21).

Starting Position: Lie on your back, left knee bent, right shin crossing the left leg.

Movement: Lift the left foot off the floor. Repeat on the left side.

Tip: Do not cross the ankle over the leg, as this may stretch the ligaments of the ankle joint.

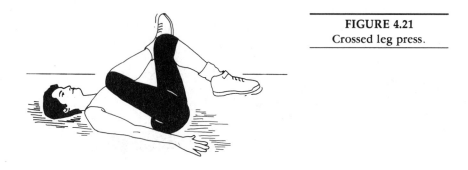

FIGURE 4.21
Crossed leg press.

Body Part: Calf

EXERCISE: Toe pull (Figure 4.22).

Starting Position: In a seated position with the knees bent, place the right heel on top of the toes of the left foot. Grasp the toes of the right foot with the right hand.

Movement: Slowly extend the legs until you experience mild tension. Repeat on the left side.

Tip: Avoid leaning over to reach the toes. Do not lock the knee of the extended leg.

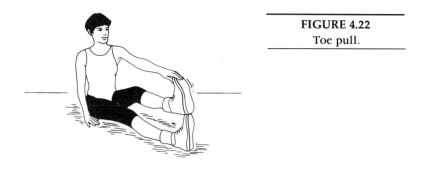

FIGURE 4.22
Toe pull.

Body Part: Front of Thigh

EXERCISE: Lying heel pull (Figure 4.23).

Starting Position: Lying on your stomach, hold the right foot with the right hand, keeping both legs together and pointed straight back.

Movement: Pull the right foot toward the buttocks. For greater stretch, press the hips into the floor. Repeat on the left side.

Tips: Do not arch the back and do not pull the knee upward off the floor or out to the side. Discontinue this exercise if it hurts your knee. If you cannot reach your foot without taking your head and shoulders off the floor or without pulling your knee out to the side, place a towel around your ankle and gently pull on the towel (Figure 4.24).

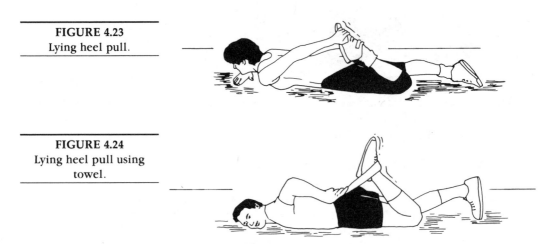

FIGURE 4.23
Lying heel pull.

FIGURE 4.24
Lying heel pull using
towel.

Body Part: Chest and Shoulders

EXERCISE: Lying underarm press (Figure 4.25).

Starting Position: Lie on your stomach, forehead on the floor. Grasp both hands behind your back, bending the elbows slightly.

Movement: Gently press the arms upward.

Tip: Keep the elbows bent.

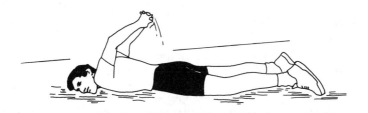

FIGURE 4.25
Lying underarm press.

Sample Post Stretch Routine

Sequence	Counts	Body Position	Flexibility Exercise
1	32	Sitting	Overarm press
2	32	Sitting with legs extended	Toe pull (right side)
Repeat sequence 2 on the left side			
3	4	Sitting with knees bent	Curl down to the floor
4	32	Lying on back	Knees to chest
5	32	Lying on back	Leg pull (right side)
Repeat sequence 5 on the left side			
6	8	Lying on back	Knees to chest
7	32	Lying on back	Straddle
8	32	Lying on back	Crossed leg press (right side)
Repeat sequence 8 on the left side			
9	32	Lying on abdomen	Lying heel pull (right side)
Repeat sequence 9 on the left side			
10	32	Lying on abdomen	Lying underarm press
11	32	Kneeling	Diagonal arm pull (right side)
Repeat sequence 11 on the left side			
12	32	Standing	Elbow press (right side)
Repeat sequence 12 on the left side			

Risky Stretching Exercises

The following exercises are considered to be potentially hazardous because they place excessive stress on specific joints of the body. They generally should be avoided.

Exercises: Unsupported forward flexion in a standing position (Figure 4.26)
Unsupported forward flexion in a standing position with a twisting motion (Figure 4.27)

Danger: These positions place uneven compression on the intervertebral discs of the lower spine and could result in a back injury.

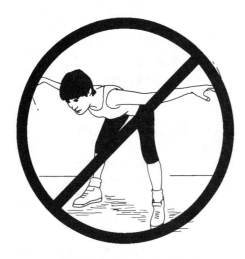

FIGURE 4.26
Unsupported forward
flexion.

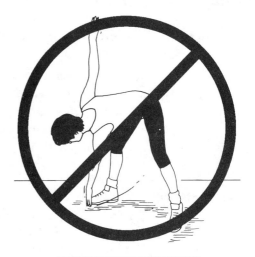

FIGURE 4.27
Unsupported forward
flexion with a twisting
motion.

Exercises: Neck hyperextension (Figure 4.28)
Yoga plough (Figure 4.29)

Danger: These exercise positions place excessive stress on the intervertebral discs of the upper spine and could result in a neck injury.

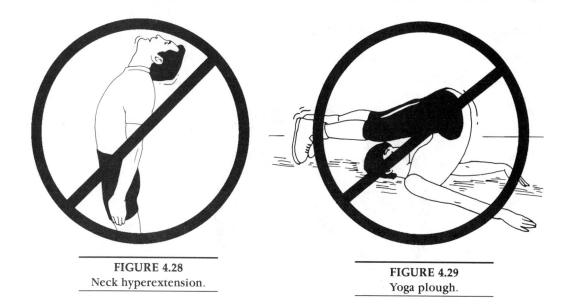

FIGURE 4.28
Neck hyperextension.

FIGURE 4.29
Yoga plough.

Exercises: Hurdler stretch (Figure 4.30)
Loaded deep knee flexion (Figure 4.31)

Danger: These exercises can stretch the ligaments surrounding the knee and could result in a knee injury.

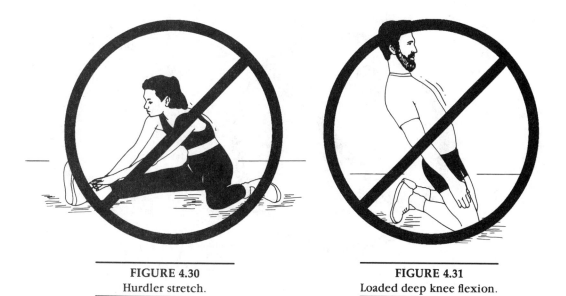

FIGURE 4.30
Hurdler stretch.

FIGURE 4.31
Loaded deep knee flexion.

Exercise: Hyperextending the joints (Figure 4.32)

Danger: Frequent hyperextension of a joint can cause the ligaments to stretch, destabilizing the joint.

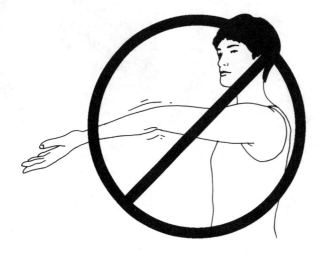

FIGURE 4.32
Hyperextending the joints.

Exercise: Fast circling of a limb, the trunk, or the head (Figure 4.33)

Danger: Uncontrolled circling can cause serious damage to the spine or the joint.

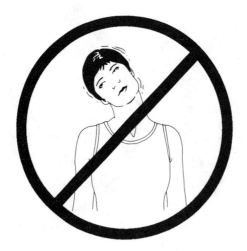

FIGURE 4.33
Fast circling of a limb, the trunk, or the head.

KEY POINTS IN CHAPTER 4

1. Flexibility is the range of possible motion at each joint and is usually limited by tight muscles.

2. Flexibility exercises enhance personal appearance and exercise performance and reduce the risk of developing joint-related injuries caused by tight muscles.

3. Static stretching is the safest method for improving flexibility.

4. Always warm up for three to five minutes before stretching.

5. Stretch before and after aerobic activity.

6. Hold each stretch for at least ten seconds.

7. Stretch to the point of tension, not pain.

8. Discontinue any stretching exercises that cause undue pain and discomfort. Consult your instructor.

9. Avoid hazardous stretching exercises and positions.

5 Muscular Strength and Endurance

TEST YOUR KNOWLEDGE

Answer true or false to the following statements:

1. The best way to reduce the fat surrounding your waist is to regularly perform abdominal exercises. True False

   Answer: False. You cannot selectively remove fat from one area of your body by performing a specific exercise for a particular body part.

2. Exercising a muscle until it burns is an ideal technique for strengthening and firming that muscle. True False

   Answer: False. Although "going for the burn" increases muscular endurance, it does not significantly improve strength and it can result in an injury.

3. Women who lift heavy weights will develop bulging muscles. True False

   Answer: False. Most women do not have enough of the hormone testosterone to develop bulging muscles.

4. Leg-lowering exercises are excellent for improving abdominal strength. True False

   Answer: False. Leg-lowering exercises tend to strengthen the psoas muscle (a hip flexor) rather than the abdominals. For most people, these exercises place excessive stress on the lower back region.

Principles of Muscular Strength and Endurance

Muscular strength is the maximum amount of force that can be exerted by a muscle against resistance. A strength exercise is one that causes the muscle to contract against some external force. Regular participation in a resistance training program will cause the muscle fibers to enlarge or *hypertrophy*.

Two types of muscular contractions occur when you perform a resistance exercise such as a sit-up. The shortening phase against resistance is called a *concentric contraction,* and the lengthening phase is called an *eccentric contraction*. Lifting the head, shoulders, and back off the floor during a curl-up is an example of a concentric contraction of the abdominal muscles (muscles are shortening); lowering the trunk onto the floor results in an eccentric contraction of the abdominal muscles (muscles are lengthening). The concentric and eccentric phases of a resistance exercise are equally important. For example, when lifting a heavy object such as a television set, you not only need arm strength to lift the TV (concentric contraction of the biceps) but you also require arm strength to carefully lower the TV so that you don't drop it (eccentric contraction of the biceps). In most instances, it is wise to strengthen a muscle through its full range of motion because many activities require that a muscle be strong throughout its full range. For example, the gastrocnemius (calf muscle) must be strong through a wide range of movement to propel your body off the floor during high-impact movements and to control the impacts when you land.

When a muscle remains the same length while it is contracting, the contraction is *isometric*. Because no movement is taking place, isometric contractions are also called *static* contractions. Tightening your abdominals throughout the day is an example of an isometric contraction. In fact, good spinal alignment is partly maintained through a series of isometric contractions.

The ability of the muscle to repeatedly contract against resistance over an extended time period is called *muscular endurance*. Muscular endurance is particularly important for activities that require prolonged contraction of the muscles, such as performing aerobic dance for thirty minutes, carrying a heavy load up several flights of stairs, or holding your shoulders back throughout the day.

The Importance of Muscular Strength and Endurance

Muscular strength and endurance are important for maintaining proper spinal alignment, for improving appearance, and for enhancing the performance of daily activities and exercises.

Good posture is maintained when the strength of the muscles on both sides of a joint is balanced. When one muscle is much stronger than its opposing muscle, the joint tends to be pulled into a mechanically vulnerable position. For example, if the chest muscles are considerably stronger than the upper back muscles, the shoulders are pulled forward. If the muscles of the lower back and the front of the hips are stronger than the abdominal muscles, a swayback posture is adopted, placing excessive stress on the spine. A well-designed strength program will minimize muscle imbalances.

Because strong muscles help you maintain appropriate posture, they enhance your personal appearance. Strength exercises also improve muscle definition, or the shape of your muscles. Muscle definition depends on the degree of muscle hypertrophy (enlargement of the muscle fibers) and the amount of subcutaneous fat (fat under the skin) covering the muscle. To some extent, muscle definition is genetic. You can, however, increase muscular hypertrophy by regularly performing strength exercises, and you can reduce your percentage of body fat by increasing your levels of physical activity.

Muscular strength and endurance also can greatly improve your performance of daily tasks and physical activities. For example, it is easier to carry heavy objects when the muscles of the arms are strong. With enhanced muscular endurance, you can perform physical activities such as aerobic dance for longer periods of time.

Myths about Strength

1. **Myth:** When you begin exercising, fat turns into muscle, and when you stop exercising, muscle turns into fat.

   Fact: Muscle and fat are two entirely different tissues. They do not look alike and they do not serve the same function. Muscle can no more change into fat than your skin can turn into bone. Why is this misconception common? When sedentary people begin exercising, they often burn calories at a higher rate, thus reducing their total percentage of body fat. At the same time, the working muscles become firmer and more shapely. When these same people stop exercising, their muscles atrophy and they again store a higher percentage of body fat.

2. **Myth:** You can spot-reduce body fat. For example, many people perform hundreds of sit-ups a day in the hopes of reducing the fat around their hips.

   Fact: The efforts of those who try to spot-reduce are wasteful and no doubt frustrating. Unfortunately, no amount of spot exercising will selectively remove the fat from only one area of the body. Fat is metabolized from all over the body. To reduce your percentage of body fat, you must increase your level of physical activity to raise the rate at which you burn calories.

3. **Myth:** "Going for the burn" will firm muscle.

   Fact: This practice involves doing many repetitions of an exercise to the point at which the muscle experiences a burning sensation. Too many repetitions results in a buildup of waste products and a lack of oxygen, as indicated by the burning sensation. There is no research evidence to suggest that exercising while the muscle is burning will significantly strengthen or firm the muscle. There is, however, some danger of sustaining a joint injury. When people continue to exercise a muscle that is clearly fatigued (as indicated by the burning sensation), other structures, such as tendons and ligaments, become compromised.

4. **Myth:** Women who lift weights will develop bulging muscles.

   Fact: The hormone testosterone is responsible for muscle bulk. Most women have a limited amount of this hormone. Weight training for women will usually produce a smooth, sculptured look. There is no better way to develop muscular strength and definition than to use progressively heavier resistance with fewer repetitions.

Overload and Progressive Resistance

Your muscles can only get stronger when they are challenged to work harder than they are accustomed to working. This concept, called the *overload principle,* states that when a muscle is subjected to a greater-than-normal load, it will adapt by becoming stronger. For example, if you choose to perform twelve repetitions of a strength exercise, you must find the amount of weight or rubber resistance that you can lift or pull against twelve times only. In other words, the muscle should be fatigued when you complete twelve repetitions. If you can perform thirteen or more repetitions, the resistance is insufficient. Once the muscles have adapted to this load (when you can easily lift the weight or pull the rubber band twelve times), the muscles will maintain that level of strength or endurance as long as the load is not changed. To further increase muscular strength, a slightly heavier load must be used. Gradually and systematically increasing the workload is called *progressive resistance.*

The Specific Nature of Strength

Because muscular strength and endurance are specific, you must first determine which muscles you want to target and whether you wish to develop muscular strength, muscular endurance, or both. To improve strength, you need to lift more resistance a fewer number of times (six to ten repetitions). If you want to increase muscular endurance, you must lift lighter weights a greater number of times (twelve to twenty repetitions). To improve both muscular strength and endurance, it is necessary to perform at least one set of eight to twelve repetitions at least twice a week. A *set* is a group of repetitions, whereas *repetitions* are the number of times the weight is lifted consecutively.

Types of Resistance

Improvements in strength are determined by the intensity of overload, not by the technique being employed. In other words, the overload can be applied using pulleys, springs, rubber bands, tubing, or weights. For deconditioned individuals, the weight of an arm or leg may be sufficient resistance at the start of their strength program. As greater resistance is required, weights or rubber resistance can be introduced.

Muscle Imbalances

Most aerobic dance routines tend to strengthen specific muscles on one side of the joint but do little for the opposing muscle group. To prevent a muscle imbalance during aerobic dance, it is important that time be spent during the isolation work to strengthen the neglected muscles. Refer to Table 5.1 to determine which muscles require special attention during floor work.

Table 5.1   Balancing Muscle Groups

Muscles Strengthened during Aerobic Dance	Opposing Muscles Requiring Strengthening during Isolation Work*
Gastrocnemius and soleus (calf)	Tibialis anterior (shin)
Erector spinae (back) and hip flexors	Abdominals
Pectoralis major (chest)	Rhomboids and trapezius (upper back)

* For a description of specific strength exercises, see "Strength Exercises for Muscle Balance" beginning on p. 57.

Strength Guidelines

1. Wear comfortable, nonconstricting clothing.
2. Warm up and stretch before performing strength exercises. This will increase body temperature and flexibility, improving your performance and minimizing the risk of injury.
3. Perform strength exercises slowly and precisely. Poor technique can result in injury.
4. Do not fling weights. The force generated at a joint by a swinging weight can be many times greater than the actual poundage of the weight.
5. Select the type (weights or bands) and the appropriate amount of resistance.
6. Choose the appropriate number of sets and repetitions. For most exercises in an aerobic dance class, you will perform one set of eight to twelve repetitions. Remember that to adequately challenge the muscle, you must find the amount of resistance that fatigues the muscle in eight to twelve repetitions. If the muscle is not fatigued, the resistance is too light.
7. For general health, select resistance exercises for each of the major muscle groups of the body.

8. Control each exercise. For example, take 2 counts to shorten the muscle (concentric contraction), hold for 2 counts, then take 4 counts to lengthen the muscle (eccentric contractions).

9. Do not hold your breath. Breathe on each repetition.

10. If using more than one set per exercise, execute the first set for each exercise before performing a second or third set. This gives muscles adequate time to recover from strenuous exercise. For example, perform one set of abdominal curls, side leg lifts, and hamstring curls. Repeat the sequence a second and third time.

11. Give exercising muscles a day of rest between resistance training sessions.

12. Never lock the joints in full extension. This can stretch the ligaments and destabilize the joint.

13. Do not do strength training without your doctor's approval if you are pregnant or have high blood pressure, arthritis, or a major joint disorder.

14. Do not perform any strength exercises that cause unusual pain or discomfort. Consult your instructor or physician.

Guidelines for Using Rubber Bands

Rubber resistance bands are a convenient and inexpensive method for developing muscular strength. Remember that your muscles must be subjected to a greater-than-normal workload (overload principle) to develop muscular strength and definition. For a safe and effective workout with rubber resistance bands, carefully follow the strength guidelines from the preceding section and the rubber band guidelines that follow:

1. Only use bands that have been specifically designed for strength training. The bands accompanying this book are manufactured by SPRI Products for the purpose of resistance training.

2. Before each workout, check your bands for tears, punctures, or cracking. Replace defective or worn bands (see the band order form in the back of this book).

3. Maintain proper spinal alignment at all times.

4. Never hyperextend a joint. When holding a band in your hand, always keep the hand and forearm in a straight line [Figure 5.1 (a) and (b)].

5. Be sure that the line of pull on the band is never directly towards your eyes [Figure 5.2 (a) and (b)].

6. Keep repetitions smooth and controlled. With each repetition, slowly lengthen the band as far as possible, then slowly resist the tension as the band shortens.

7. Beginners should completely release the tension in the bands between each repetition, whereas the experienced exercisers may choose to maintain some tension in the band between repetitions.

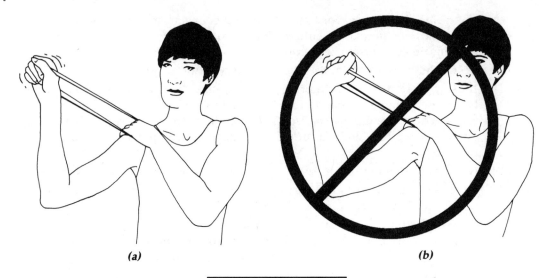

(a)   *(b)*

FIGURE 5.1
(a) Proper wrist position
with band. *(b)* Improper
wrist position.

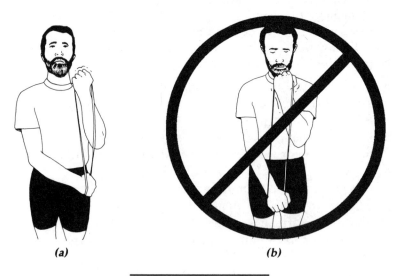

(a)   *(b)*

FIGURE 5.2
(a) Correct position—
line of pull of band away
from eyes. *(b)* Incorrect
position—line of pull of
band toward eyes.

---

8. Choose the appropriate resistance. The thicker or shorter the band, the greater the resistance. If you wish to increase the resistance, choose a thicker band or shorten the band by wrapping it more than once around your hand, ankle, or leg.

9. When using the bands on your legs, you will probably find it more comfortable to place the band over fabric such as tights, warm-up pants, or socks. If you experience discomfort on your hands, you may wish to wear gloves.

10. If you feel pain in a joint, reduce the tension in the band (choose a longer or thinner band). If the pain persists, discontinue the exercise and consult your instructor.

Strength Exercises

Perform the strength exercises for muscle balance during each aerobic dance class. Unless otherwise instructed, perform one set of eight to twelve repetitions for each exercise. Major muscles of the body are identified in Figure 5.3 (a) and (b). A sample strength routine follows the description of the exercises.

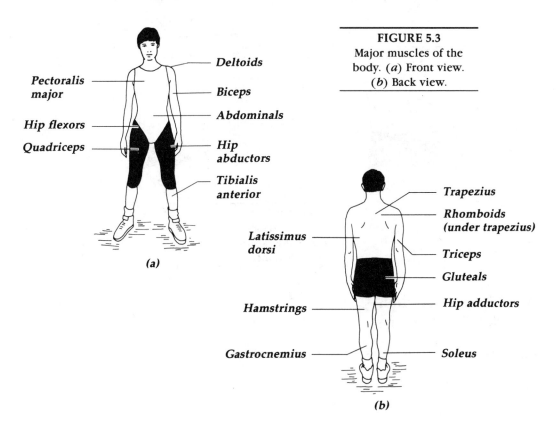

FIGURE 5.3
Major muscles of the body. (*a*) Front view. (*b*) Back view.

Deltoids
Pectoralis major
Biceps
Abdominals
Hip flexors
Quadriceps
Hip abductors
Tibialis anterior

(a)

Trapezius
Rhomboids (under trapezius)
Latissimus dorsi
Triceps
Gluteals
Hip adductors
Hamstrings
Gastrocnemius
Soleus

(b)

Body Part: Upper Back
Muscles: Rhomboids and Trapezius

EXERCISE: Elbow presses [Figure 5.4 (a) and (b)].

Equipment: Rubber band.

Starting Position: Stand or sit. Grasp the rubber band with both hands at chest level, elbows at shoulder height, palms towards you.

Movement: Pull the band apart as your elbows press back and you squeeze your shoulder blades together. Release.

Tip: Keep the elbows at shoulder height.

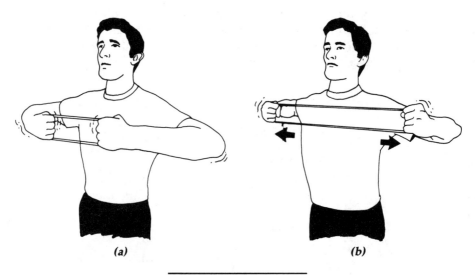

(a) (b)

FIGURE 5.4
Elbow presses.
(*a*) Starting position.
(*b*) Movement.

Body Part: Midsection
Muscles: Abdominals

EXERCISE: Pelvic tilts [Figures 5.5, 5.6, and 5.7, (a) and (b)].

Equipment: None.

Starting Position: Stand, kneel on hands and knees, or lie on the back.

Movement: Flatten your back by tightly tucking the buttocks under the hips and forcefully contracting the abdominal muscles. Hold for 8 counts. Release and repeat eight to twelve times.

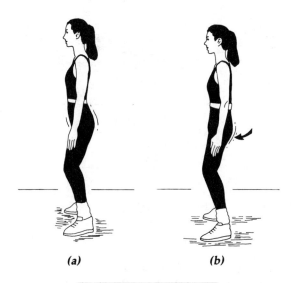

(a)   **(b)**

FIGURE 5.5
Standing pelvic tilts.
(*a*) Starting position.
(*b*) Movement.

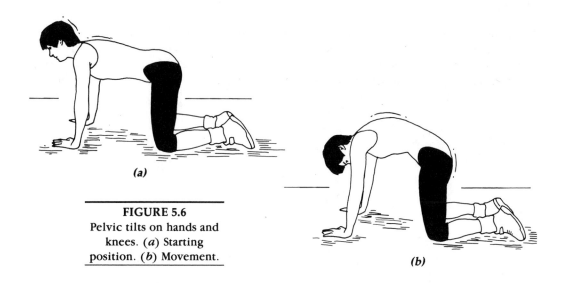

(a)

FIGURE 5.6
Pelvic tilts on hands and knees. (*a*) Starting position. (*b*) Movement.

(b)

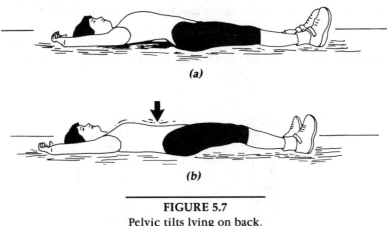

FIGURE 5.7
Pelvic tilts lying on back.
(*a*) Starting position.
(*b*) Movement.

EXERCISE: Curl-ups [Figure 5.8 (a) and (b)].

Equipment: None.

Starting Position: Lie on the back, feet flat, knees bent or knees to chest, and hands cupped at the base of the head. Press the back flat to the floor.

Movement: Curl the head and upper back off the floor and curl back down. Take 4 counts to curl up and 4 counts to curl down. Repeat twelve times. To add greater resistance, curl up 4 counts, hold for 4 or 8 counts, then curl down for 4 counts. Repeat eight to twelve times.

Tips: Move smoothly and continuously. Do not initiate the upward movement with the head or arms. Contract the abdominal muscles to create the movement. Use the hands behind the neck to support the weight of the head, minimizing the need for muscular contraction of the neck muscles. Keep the lower back firmly pressed against the floor as you curl up and down.

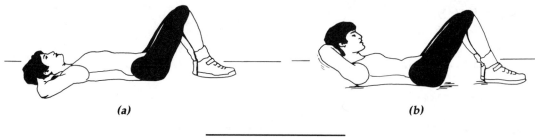

FIGURE 5.8
Curl ups. (*a*) Starting
postion. (*b*) Movement.

EXERCISE: Diagonal curl [Figure 5.9 (a) and (b)].

Equipment: None.

Starting Position: Lie on your back with the left shin crossed over the right leg, hands cupped at the base of the head.

Movement: Curl the head and upper back upward on count 1, twist the trunk and right elbow toward the left knee on count 2, twist back to center on count 3, and curl back down to the floor on count 4. Perform eight to twelve repetitions on each side.

Tips: Keep your lower back on the floor. Be sure to twist from the waist and not just from the shoulders.

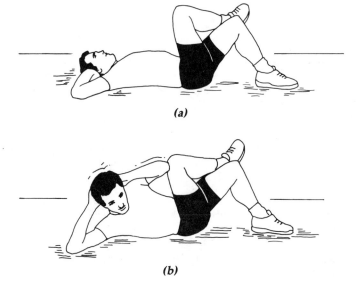

FIGURE 5.9
Diagonal curl.
(*a*) Starting position.
(*b*) Movement.

(a)

(b)

Body Part: Shins
Muscles: Tibialis Anterior

EXERCISE: Toe taps [Figure 5.10 (a) and (b)].

Equipment: None.

Starting Position: Stand with the feet shoulder-width apart.

Movement: Leaving your heel on the floor, vigorously tap your right foot up and down. After eight to twelve repetitions, repeat with the left foot.

Tip: Do not hyperextend the knee joint.

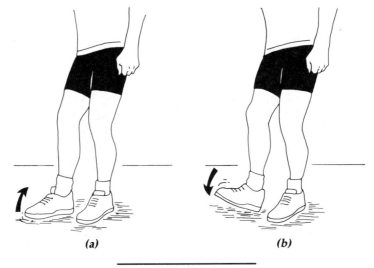

(a) (b)

FIGURE 5.10
Toe taps. (*a*) Starting
position. (*b*) Movement.

EXERCISE: Foot curls [Figure 5.11 (a) and (b)].

Equipment: Rubber band.

Starting Position: Sit with a rubber band across both feet. Extend the left leg to the front, holding the right knee toward your chest with the right foot slightly flexed.

Movement: Pull your toes up toward your knees, then point your toes. After eight to twelve repetitions, repeat on the left foot.

Tips: Be sure that there is enough tension on the band to create adequate resistance. Move only the right foot; do not move at the hip or knee joint. Be sure that the line of pull on your band is not in the direction of your eyes or someone else's eyes.

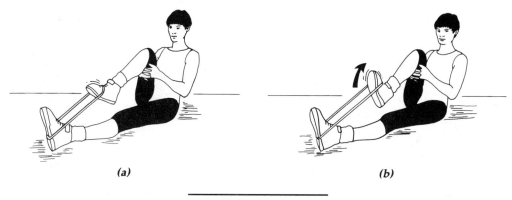

(a)   *(b)*

FIGURE 5.11
Foot curls. (*a*) Starting
position. (*b*) Movement.

If you have additional class time, select among the specific strength exercises that follow. Unless otherwise indicated, perform one set of eight to twelve repetitions on the right side before repeating the exercise on the left side.

Body Part: Front of Upper Arms
Muscles: Biceps

EXERCISE: Arm curls [Figure 5.12 (a) and (b)].

Equipment: Rubber band.

Starting Position: Stand or sit, holding the band with the left palm down and the right palm up. Secure the band against the right hip with the left hand.

Movement: Keeping the right elbow against the body, pull the band upward towards the right shoulder. Release. After eight to twelve repetitions, repeat on the left side.

Tips: Do not hyperextend the wrist. To increase tension, drop the lower hand further down the hip.

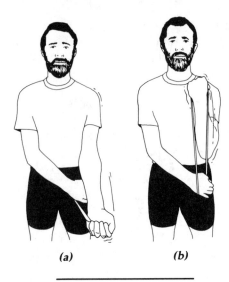

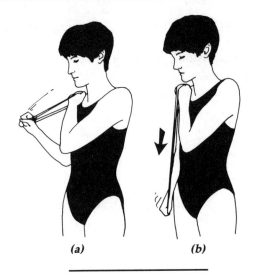

FIGURE 5.12
Arm curls. (*a*) Starting
position. (*b*) Movement.

FIGURE 5.13
Downward elbow
extensions. (*a*) Starting
position. (*b*) Movement.

Body Part: Back of Upper Arms
Muscles: Triceps

EXERCISE: Downward elbow extensions [Figure 5.13 (a) and (b)].

Equipment: Rubber band.

Starting Position: Stand or sit with the left hand through the top of the band and on the right shoulder, right hand through the bottom of the band, palm facing down.

Movement: With the right elbow at the side of the body, press the right hand down toward the hips. Release. After eight to twelve repetitions, repeat on the left side.

Tip: Do not hyperextend the wrist.

EXERCISE: Upward elbow extensions [Figure 5.14 (a) and (b)].

Equipment: Rubber band.

Starting Position: Stand or sit with the left hand through the bottom of the band and on the right shoulder, right hand through top of the band, palm facing up.

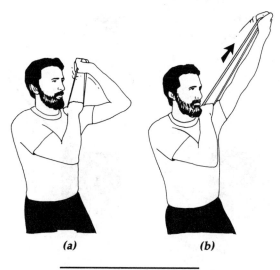

(a) **(b)**

FIGURE 5.14
Upward elbow
extensions. (*a*) Starting
position. (*b*) Movement.

Movement: Press the right hand overhead. Release. After eight to twelve repetitions, repeat on the left side.

Tip: Do not hyperextend the wrist or the elbow.

Body Part: Top of the Shoulders
Muscles: Deltoids

EXERCISE: Front shoulder raises [Figure 5.15 (a) and (b)].

Equipment: Rubber band.

Starting Position: Stand and hold the band with both hands in front of the right hip.

Movement: Keep the left hand in front of the right hip and lift the right arm forward and up to shoulder height. Release. After eight to twelve repetitions, repeat on the left side.

Tips: Do not hyperextend the elbow joints. If you experience discomfort in the shoulder joint, use a longer band or bend the elbow slightly.

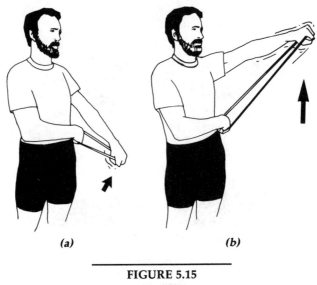

FIGURE 5.15
Front shoulder raises.
(*a*) Starting position.
(*b*) Movement.

EXERCISE: Side shoulder raises [Figure 5.16 (a) and (b)].

Equipment: Rubber band.

Starting Position: Stand while grasping the top of the band with the right hand. Holding the band behind the back and against the right side, grasp the bottom of the band with the left hand.

Movement: Lift the right arm up to the side to shoulder height. Release. After eight to twelve repetitions, repeat on the left side.

Tips: Do not hyperextend the elbows. If you experience discomfort in the shoulder joint, use a longer band or bend the elbow slightly.

Body Part: Chest
Muscles: Pectoralis Major

EXERCISE: Chest crosses [Figure 5.17 (a) and (b)].

Equipment: Rubber band.

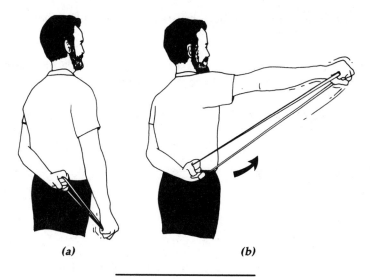

FIGURE 5.16
Side shoulder raises.
(*a*) Starting position.
(*b*) Movement.

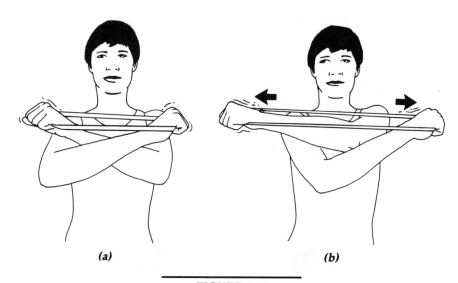

FIGURE 5.17
Chest crosses. (*a*) Starting
position. (*b*) Movement.

Starting Position: Stand or sit with both hands through the band, hands crossed, palms facing away from each other.

Movement: Press the hands apart and release. Alternate the right hand over the left and the left hand over the right. Repeat eight to twelve times.

Tip: Do not hyperextend the wrist.

Body Part: Back
Muscles: Latissimus Dorsi

EXERCISE: Lat pull downs [Figure 5.18 (a) and (b)].

Equipment: Rubber band.

Starting Position: Stand or sit, grasping the band with both hands, palms facing each other, band above the head.

Movement: Pull the elbow downward. Release. After eight to twelve repetitions, repeat on the other side.

Tip: Do not hyperextend the elbows.

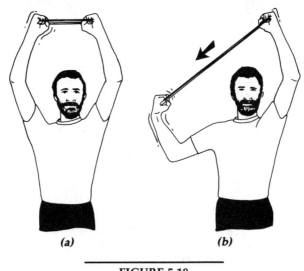

(a)   *(b)*

FIGURE 5.18
Lat pull downs.
(*a*) Starting position.
(*b*) Movement.

Body Part: Front of Hips
Muscles: Hip Flexors

EXERCISE: Front leg raise [Figure 5.19 (a) and (b)].

Equipment: Rubber band.

Starting Position: Sit with both legs extended in front and the ankles crossed. Place the band under the left foot and around the right ankle.

Movement: Lift the right leg upward. Release. After eight to twelve repetitions, repeat with the left leg.

Tip: Do not hyperextend the knees.

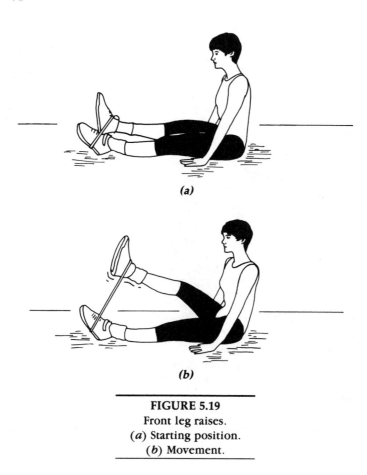

(a)

(b)

FIGURE 5.19
Front leg raises.
(*a*) Starting position.
(*b*) Movement.

Body Part: Front of Thighs
Muscles: Quadriceps

EXERCISE: Knee extensions [Figure 5.20 (a) and (b)].

Equipment: Rubber band.

Starting Position: Sit with the knees bent and the ankles crossed. Place the band under the left foot and around the right ankle.

Movement: Extend the knee, lifting the right foot upwards. Release. After eight to twelve repetitions, repeat on the left leg.

Tip: Do not hyperextend the knees at the end of the movement.

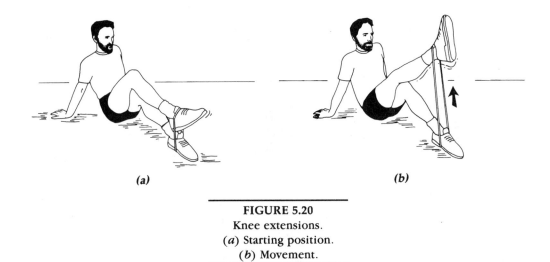

(a)   **(b)**

FIGURE 5.20
Knee extensions.
(*a*) Starting position.
(*b*) Movement.

Body Part: Outer Thighs
Muscles: Hip Abductors

EXERCISE: Outer thigh lift [Figure 5.21 (a) and (b)].

Equipment: Rubber band.

Starting Position: Lie on the left side, left knee slightly bent for support, right leg straight and band around both shins.

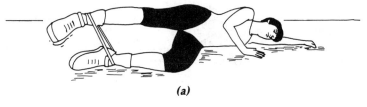

(a)

FIGURE 5.21
Outer thigh lifts.
(*a*) Starting position.
(*b*) Movement.

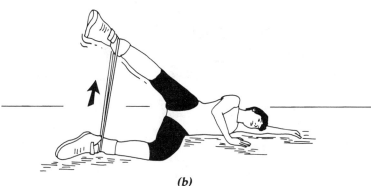

(b)

Movement: Keeping the foot, knee, and thigh facing forward, lift the right leg. Release. After eight to twelve repetitions, repeat on the left leg.

Tips: Do not hyperextend the back. Do not turn the leg upward or you will be working the hip flexors. Do not bend the right leg at the hip (L position). If the band feels too tight or you feel tension in the knee joint, place the band slightly above or below the knee.

Body Part: Inner Thighs
Muscles: Hip Adductors

EXERCISE: Inner thigh lift [Figure 5.22 (a) and (b)].

Equipment: Rubber band.

Starting Position: Lie on the left side, right foot and knee on the floor in front of the left leg, left leg straight, band around the left shin and under the right foot.

Movement: Keeping the foot, knee, and thigh facing forward, lift the left leg. Release. After eight to twelve repetitions, repeat on the right leg.

Tips: Do not hyperextend the back. Do not turn the leg upward or you will be working the hip flexors. If the band feels too tight or you feel tension in the knee joint, place the band slightly above or below the knee.

FIGURE 5.22
Inner thigh lifts.
(*a*) Starting position.
(*b*) Movement.

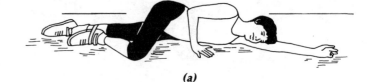

(a)

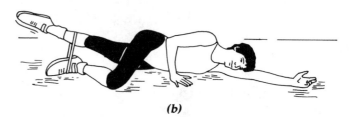

(b)

Body Part: Back of Thigh
Muscles: Hamstrings

EXERCISE: Leg curls [Figure 5.23 (a) and (b)].

Equipment: Rubber band.

Starting Position: Lie on your abdomen, head and shoulders down, band around the left ankle and across the right foot, ankles crossed.

Movement: Curl the right foot toward the buttock. Release. After eight to twelve repetitions, repeat on the left leg.

Tip: Do not hyperextend the back.

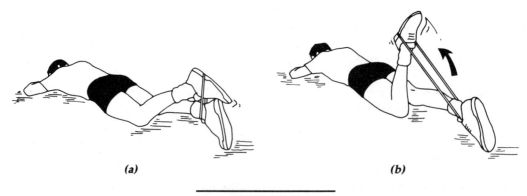

(a)   **(b)**

FIGURE 5.23
Leg curls. (*a*) Starting
position. (*b*) Movement.

Sample Strength Routine

Sequence	Body Position	Strength Exercise	Sets/Repetitions
1	Seated	Elbow presses	1/12
2	Seated	Lat pull downs	1/12 (right and left)
3	Seated	Foot curls	1/12 (right and left)
4	Lying on back	Curl ups	1/12
5	Lying on left side	Outer thigh lift	1/12 (right only)
6	Lying on left side	Inner thigh lift	1/12 (left only)
7	Lying on abdomen	Leg curls	1/12 (right then left)
8	Lying on back	Diagonal curls	1/12 (right and left)
9	Lying on right side	Outer thigh lift	1/12 (left only)
10	Lying on right side	Inner thigh lift	1/12 (right only)

Risky Strength Exercises

The following strength exercises can potentially injure your musculoskeletal system. Avoid these exercises whenever possible.

Exercises: Single or double leg lowering (Figure 5.24)
Straight-legged sit-ups (Figure 5.25)
Back hyperextension (Figure 5.26)
Standing and bending forward while holding weights (Figure 5.27)

Danger: All of these exercises place tremendous stress on the intervertebral discs of the lumbar spine and could result in a lower back injury.

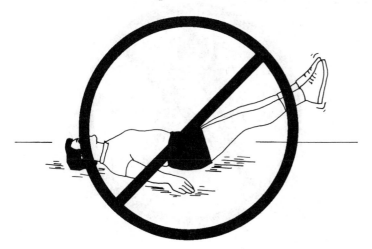

FIGURE 5.24
Single or double leg lowering.

FIGURE 5.25
Straight-legged sit-ups.

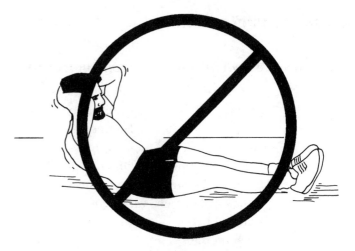

FIGURE 5.26
Back hyperextension.

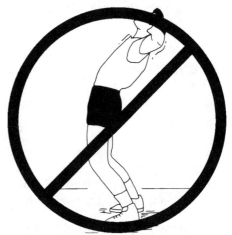

FIGURE 5.27
Standing and bending
forward while holding
weights.

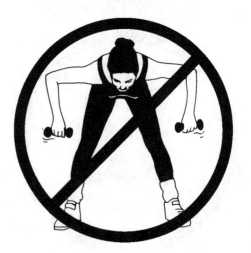

Exercise: Deep knee bends or full squats (Figure 5.28)

Danger: Full squats place an enormous amount of stress on the ligaments and the cartilage of the knee joint and could cause a serious knee injury.

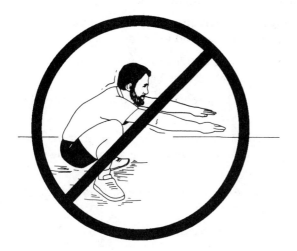

FIGURE 5.28
Deep knee bends or full squats.

Exercise: Hyperextending the knees or elbows while holding weights (Figure 5.29)

Danger: These exercise positions stretch the ligaments surrounding the joint and could result in an injury.

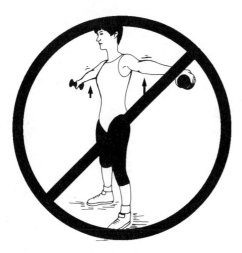

FIGURE 5.29
Hyperextending the knees or elbows while holding weights.

KEY POINTS IN CHAPTER 5

1. Muscular strength is the maximum amount of force exerted by a muscle against resistance; muscular endurance is the ability of a muscle to repeatedly contract against resistance over an extended period of time.

2. Muscular strength and endurance are important for maintaining proper spinal alignment, improving appearance, and enhancing performance.

3. To increase muscular strength or endurance, the muscle must be overloaded using techniques of progressive resistance.

4. Muscle imbalances can be avoided by strengthening the muscles on both sides of a joint.

5. To improve muscular endurance and strength, perform at least one set of eight to twelve repetitions of exercises for each of the major muscle groups at least twice a week.

6. Discontinue any exercise that causes undue pain or discomfort. Consult your instructor.

7. Avoid strength exercises and positions that are potentially hazardous.

6 *Achieving Aerobic Fitness*

TEST YOUR KNOWLEDGE

Answer true or false to the following statements:

1. If you are thin, you are aerobically fit.   True   False

   Answer: False. It is possible to be thin and have a very low level of aerobic fitness, especially if you do not perform any aerobic activity.

2. The more quickly your exercise heart rate recovers back toward resting levels, the better your aerobic fitness.   True   False

   Answer: True. The lower your recovery heart rate following exercise, the better your aerobic fitness.

3. To achieve maximum health, it is important that your aerobic dance activity be as intense as you can tolerate.   True   False

   Answer: False. Extremely high intensities of exercise can result in musculoskeletal injury.

4. The best way to improve your aerobic fitness is to simultaneously increase the exercise intensity, the length of each exercise session, and the number of times you exercise each week.   True   False

   Answer: False. Although a simultaneous increase in exercise intensity, duration, and frequency will improve aerobic fitness, it will also greatly increase your risk of injury. To allow your body adequate time for adaptation, it is best to change only one variable at a time.

Principles and Importance of Aerobic Fitness

Aerobic fitness, also called *cardiovascular* or *cardiorespiratory endurance,* is the ability of the heart and lungs to deliver oxygen to the working muscles during sustained movement. Breathlessness and exhaustion are usually experienced when there is an insufficient amount of blood pumped to the working muscles during moderate to strenuous exercise. Increasing your level of aerobic fitness enhances your heart's ability to pump adequate amounts of oxygenated blood to the working muscles, allowing you to perform prolonged exercise with less fatigue.

Aerobic activities that improve cardiovascular endurance use the large muscles of the body vigorously and continuously over an extended time period (usually twenty minutes or more). Aerobic dance is an excellent aerobic activity.

The benefits of regular participation in aerobic exercise include (1) improved efficiency of your heart and lungs, allowing you to perform daily tasks and leisure activities with less fatigue; (2) faster recovery from strenuous exercise and daily tasks; (3) reduced risk of developing coronary heart disease; and (4) decreased body fat and increased lean body weight.

Myths about Aerobic Fitness

1. **Myth:** If you are thin, you are aerobically fit.

   Fact: Your body weight alone does not ensure that your heart, lungs, and muscles are efficient. It is possible to be thin and have poor aerobic fitness. It is also possible to look thin and have a high percentage of body fat.

2. **Myth:** A low resting heart rate is an indicator of aerobic fitness.

   Fact: Although aerobic exercise tends to lower your resting heart rate, some people are born with low resting heart rates. Unless you perform regular aerobic exercise, you are not likely to have a high level of aerobic fitness.

3. **Myth:** Weight training will not only strengthen your muscles but will also enhance your aerobic fitness.

   Fact: During resistance training, a relatively small muscle mass is activated for a brief time. To improve aerobic fitness, large volumes of blood must be pumped to the major working muscles of the body for a continuous and extended period of time. Although your exercise heart rate can increase substantially during strength training, it is most often the result of increased resistance of the blood flow back to the heart (not an increase in the amount of blood delivered to the muscles, which is necessary to improve cardiovascular endurance).

Intensity, Duration, and Frequency of Exercise

Improvements in aerobic fitness depend on the frequency (how often), duration (how long), and intensity (how hard) of exercise. Ideally, you want to optimize each of these factors to improve aerobic fitness while minimizing the risk of injury. To accomplish this goal, the following guidelines are recommended for aerobic dance:

1. Frequency—three to four times per week on alternate days;
2. Duration—twenty to thirty consecutive minutes during the aerobic portion of the class;
3. Intensity—50 to 75 percent of maximal heart-rate reserve or 60 to 80 percent of maximum heart rate (to calculate exercise intensity, see "Measuring Exercise Intensity").

Although you may achieve small gains in aerobic fitness by exceeding these guidelines, the risk of musculoskeletal injury increases considerably as you raise the intensity, duration, and frequency of exercise.

Measuring Exercise Intensity

To determine whether you are exercising at an appropriate intensity level, you will first need to calculate your target heart-rate zone. Many heart-rate charts and posters are based on the *maximal heart-rate formula*. This formula is simpler to use but is not quite as accurate as the *maximum heart-rate reserve formula*, which takes your resting heart rate (RHR) into account. To calculate *maximal heart rate*, use the following formula:

220 − Age × Percentage of training/6 = 10-second heart rate.
(60–80%)

The following is an example of a target heart-rate zone for a twenty year old using the *maximal heart-rate formula:*

60%   220 − 20 = 200 × 0.6 = 120/6 = 20.
80%   220 − 20 = 200 × 0.8 = 160/6 = 26.6, or 27.

To enhance aerobic fitness, this person's exercise heart rate following aerobic activity should be between 20 and 27 beats (ten-second count).

To calculate target heart rate using the *maximum heart-rate reserve formula,* you will need to find your resting heart rate (RHR). Place your middle and index fingers on either the carotid artery at your neck (Figure 6.1) or the radial artery on the thumb side of your wrist (Figure 6.2). Count each heart beat for one minute. It is best to find your resting pulse as soon as you wake up in the morning. Complete the following formula:

220 − Age − RHR × Percentage of training − RHR/6 = 10-second heart rate.
(50–75%)

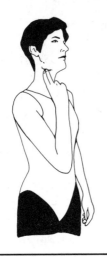

FIGURE 6.1
Checking heart rate at
carotid artery on neck.

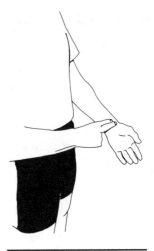

FIGURE 6.2
Checking heart rate at
radial artery on wrist.

The following is an example of a target heart-rate zone using *Karvonen's formula* for a twenty year old with a resting heart rate of 70 beats per minute:

50% $220 - 20 = 200 - 70 = 130 \times 0.5 = 65 + 70 = 135/6 = 22.5$, or 23.
75% $220 - 20 = 200 - 70 = 130 \times 0.75 = 97.5 + 70 = 167.5/6 = 27.9$, or 28.

This person's exercise heart rate should be between 23 and 28 beats (ten-second count).

On completing aerobic exercise, you should immediately locate your pulse at the carotid or radial artery. Be cautious about pressing too hard on the carotid artery, as it may cause the pulse to slow down. Count each beat for ten seconds. Compare your exercise heart rate to your target heart-rate zone.

Changing the Exercise Intensity

If you find that you are not exercising hard enough to be in your target heart-rate zone, you can increase the exercise intensity of your aerobic dance routine in the following ways:

1. Dance to faster music (although this is usually controlled by the instructor);
2. Use larger arm and leg movements;
3. Travel in various directions (forward, backwards, to the sides, diagonally, in circles);
4. Lift your feet higher off the floor (higher-impact movements);
5. Cover more distance with each step pattern.

If you decide to increase exercise intensity, be sure to change only one variable at a time. Your body needs time to adapt to the increased levels of stress. The greater the degree of change, the greater the risk of injury. For example, do not lift your feet higher off the floor if your instructor has increased the music's tempo.

Recovery Heart Rate

Recovery heart rate can be a good indicator of your current level of cardiovascular endurance. The faster your heart rate recovers to resting levels following exercise, the better your aerobic fitness. Two minutes after you have taken your exercise heart rate, take a recovery heart rate for ten seconds. Record the results. Assuming that the workload is consistent from one exercise session to another, you should notice a decrease in your recovery heart rate over time, indicating an improvement in your aerobic fitness.

Signs of Overtraining

It is possible to exercise too hard. Signs of overexercising during aerobic activity include the following complications:

1. Dizziness;
2. Severe breathlessness;
3. Nausea;
4. High heart rate;
5. Extreme fatigue;
6. Tightness in the chest.

If you experience any of these symptoms, stop exercising immediately and consult your instructor.

Environmental Considerations

A number of environmental conditions—such as high heat, high humidity, and high altitude—can adversely affect your participation in aerobic dance.

High heat and humidity are common problems during the summer months. Your body must be able to dissipate the metabolic heat produced during exercise. To reduce internal body heat, the warm blood is shunted to just below the skin surface, where it is cooled by the surrounding air and by the perspiration that forms on your skin. When the air temperature is high, sweating becomes more profuse, your body loses a considerable amount of water, and the blood returns to the heart more slowly. This could result in cardiovascular stress, which is manifested by very high heart rates.

A more stressful situation is when the heat and the humidity are both high. Perspiration must evaporate to cool the body. When the air is already saturated with moisture on humid days, your perspiration cannot evaporate, causing the sweat to roll off your skin. High humidity, therefore, impairs your body's ability to dissipate internal heat produced during exercise. Be cautious of humidity levels above 60 percent, especially when the temperature is high. Continued participation in aerobic dance when conditions are hot and humid can result in heat exhaustion or heat stroke. It is wise to discontinue or reduce the intensity of activity when weather conditions become hazardous. In addition, fluids must be more frequently replaced on hot, humid days. Drink both before and during exercise whether or not you are thirsty.

At moderate to high altitudes, an exerciser cannot deliver as much oxygen to the exercising muscles. If you normally exercise at sea level, you will need to decrease your exercise intensity at a higher altitude. You will probably experience respiratory distress and your recovery from exercise will be delayed if you try to exercise at a normal intensity. Thus, reduce exercise intensity and increase warm-up and cool-down periods until your body has adapted to this new altitude. It takes weeks to adapt to major changes in altitude.

KEY POINTS IN CHAPTER 6

1. Aerobic fitness enhances your heart's ability to pump adequate amounts of oxygenated blood to the working muscles, allowing you to perform prolonged exercise with less fatigue.

2. Regular participation in aerobic dance reduces your risk of developing heart disease by improving the efficiency of your heart and lungs and by decreasing the percentage of total body fat.

3. To improve aerobic fitness and to reduce the risk of musculoskeletal injury, the recommended guidelines for intensity, duration, and frequency of aerobic dance are twenty to thirty continuous minutes, three to four times per week on alternate days, at an intensity level of 50 to 75 percent of maximal heart-rate reserve or 60 to 80 percent of maximum heart rate.

4. Recovery heart rate taken after aerobic exercise can be used as an indicator of improved aerobic fitness.

5. If you experience signs of overtraining, stop exercising immediately and consult your instructor.

6. High heat, high humidity, and high altitude can adversely affect your aerobic dance performance. Modify your exercise routine accordingly.

7 Aerobic Dance Technique

TEST YOUR KNOWLEDGE

Answer true or false to the following statements:

1. Low-impact aerobics (LIA) is the safest form of aerobic dance for all exercise participants.　　True　　False

   Answer: False. LIA may be inappropriate for certain individuals, such as people suffering from various forms of knee discomfort.

2. To minimize the stress on the feet, knees, hips, and back during aerobic dance, it is best to significantly reduce the amount of lower body movement and increase the use of the arms.　　True　　False

   Answer: False. Since the arms have one-fourth to one-fifth of the muscle mass of the legs, they can contribute only an additional 20 to 25 percent of the work necessary to improve aerobic fitness. Therefore, the arms cannot compensate for a substantial reduction in leg movements. Use the arms for a moderate increase in exercise intensity and for variety but not as a substitute for leg work.

3. It is important to sit down on the floor immediately following the vigorous aerobic portion of your class so that your body can effectively cool down.　　True　　False

   Answer: False. To prevent pooling of blood in the legs, it is important that you remain on your feet and perform slow, rhythmic movements to help the blood return from the legs to the heart.

4. The only way you can effectively improve aerobic fitness is by performing vigorous and continuous rhythmic movements of the large muscles of the body for an extended period of time.　　True　　False

   Answer: False. It is possible to improve aerobic fitness by using discontinuous exercise techniques, such as interval training or circuit training.

Impacts

When your feet strike the floor during an aerobic dance routine, you are creating an impact. Aerobic dance classes are categorized as either high-impact aerobics (HIA), moderate-impact aerobics (MIA), low-impact aerobics (LIA), or a combination of high-, moderate-, and low-impact aerobics (combo aerobics). Most aerobic dance programs today use a combination of the various styles of impacts.

It has been suggested that the higher the vertical impact forces on your body, the greater the risk for musculoskeletal injury. Researchers have found that high-impact movements such as running and jumping can produce vertical impact forces that are twice as high as those for low-impact movements such as step touches and lunges. However, researchers have also discovered that the deep knee flexion during lateral movements characteristic of low-impact aerobics can be stressful to the knee joint. Each form of impact during aerobic dance has advantages and disadvantages. You must choose the style that is most appropriate for your individual needs.

The following is a description of each form of impact.

High-Impact Aerobics: HIA is characterized by both feet coming off the floor frequently. The feet usually form a narrow base of support (they are close together), and the body is propelled upward off the floor. The energy cost of HIA is high, as are the vertical impact forces on the body. Typical HIA step patterns include jogging, hopping, and jumping movements.

HIA is not recommended for the following individuals:

1. The deconditioned—Their musculoskeletal system is not yet ready for high impacts.
2. Pregnant women—Stress to the musculoskeletal system is increased during HIA because of the added weight during pregnancy. Also, hormonal changes cause the joints to become more lax and potentially less stable.
3. Those suffering from incontinence—The problem of a leaking bladder is aggravated when a person forcefully lands from high-impact movements.
4. Anyone susceptible to specific injuries that are caused or aggravated by high impacts—The inability to effectively absorb shock can lead to shin splints and lower back pain during high-impact movements.

Moderate-Impact Aerobics: MIA is characterized by a springing motion that occurs at the ankle joint and causes the body to lift upward to full extension, followed by a controlled lowering of the heels to the floor. Like HIA, the feet generally form a narrow base of support and the body is propelled upward. However, the feet remain on or very close to the floor most of the time. The exercise intensity is moderate to high, while the vertical impact forces are moderate. Twisting and knee lifts are examples of MIA movements.

MIA is not recommended for individuals with tight calf muscles. To lessen the vertical impact shock, it is important to allow the heels to touch the floor during each step. A person with tight calf muscles would have difficulty getting the heels to the floor.

Low-Impact Aerobics: LIA requires that one foot is firmly in contact with the floor at all times. To increase exercise intensity during LIA, deep knee flexion is necessary to move the body down and up like a pendulum in order to keep contact with the floor. The vertical impact forces are considerably less with LIA and the energy cost is moderate, depending on the individual's ability to exaggerate the foot work. Typical LIA movements include marches, step touches, and step points.

LIA is not recommended for the following individuals:

1. Those with knee discomfort—Deep knee flexion during lateral movements further aggravates knee problems.
2. Those with severely flattened or pronated feet—Lateral movements with deep knee flexion tend to produce a shifting of the knee cap toward the outer side of the knee joint and increase knee stress.
3. Those who cannot achieve target heart rate—People with a high level of aerobic fitness or individuals who do not exaggerate the foot work during LIA may find it difficult to achieve target heart rate.

When selecting a particular style of impact, choose the one that will produce the least amount of discomfort for you. Most aerobic dance steps can be modified from high-impact to moderate- or low-impact. For example, you can reduce the impacts of a jog (HIA) (Figure 7.1) by keeping the toes in contact with the floor while lifting to full extension (MIA) (Figure 7.2) or by marching vigorously while leaving one foot on the floor at all times (LIA) (Figure 7.3). If you are in a HIA class and would prefer to do LIA movements, try to modify the steps yourself.

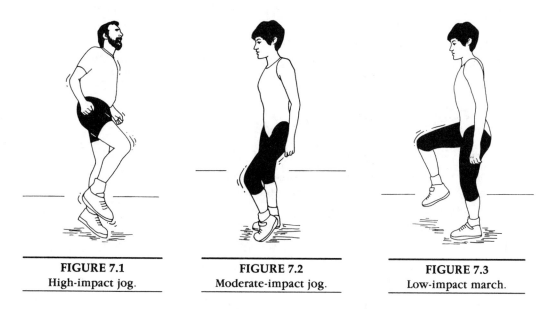

| **FIGURE 7.1** | **FIGURE 7.2** | **FIGURE 7.3** |
| High-impact jog. | Moderate-impact jog. | Low-impact march. |

Aerobic Dance Guidelines

1. Wear clothing that will not constrict your movement.
2. Warm up and pre-stretch before aerobic dancing. These activities will prepare your body for vigorous aerobic exercise, minimizing the risk of injury.
3. After the warm-up, *gradually* increase the exercise intensity. A sudden increase in the intensity of exercise could cause an abnormal heart response to exercise.
4. Perform aerobic exercise for twenty to thirty minutes in duration. If you are deconditioned, begin with ten minutes at a time, gradually progressing to thirty minutes.
5. Exercise at an intensity level equivalent to 50 to 75 percent of maximal heart-rate reserve or 60 to 80 percent of maximum heart rate.
6. Take your exercise heart rate immediately following the aerobic dance segment of your class. Count for ten seconds. Beginners should take their pulse more frequently, checking for overexertion. Your exercise heart rate should be within your target zone. If it is not, you need to make appropriate adjustments in the intensity level of your exercise.
7. Select the appropriate style of impact—HIA, MIA, LIA, or a combination.
8. Always cool down for three to five minutes following aerobic exercise. Use slow, rhythmic movements in a standing position.
9. Monitor and record your recovery heart rate after aerobic exercise. Remember, a decrease in recovery heart rate over time indicates improvements in your aerobic fitness.
10. Participate in aerobic dance classes at least three times per week but not more than four times per week on alternate days.

Aerobic Dance Precautions

Follow these recommendations to minimize the risk of injury.

1. Do not perform more than four consecutive hops on one leg at a time to minimize the musculoskeletal stress on the weight-bearing leg.
2. Avoid excessive and prolonged deep knee flexion.
3. Avoid excessive lateral movements to minimize stress on the knee joint.
4. Do not fling the limbs at any time; keep all movements controlled.
5. Do not maintain the arms at or above shoulder level for extended periods of time. This increases blood pressure (a problem for people who already have high blood pressure) and places excessive stress on the tendons and ligaments of the shoulder joint. Frequently alternate between low-, mid-, and high-range arm movements.
6. Maintain proper body alignment at all times.

7. Avoid changing directions rapidly.

8. Avoid continuous movements that require remaining on the balls of the feet for an extended period of time. Allow the heels to contact the floor as much as possible to help absorb shock.

9. When the knees are bent or flexed, make sure that the knees are centered directly over the toes.

Aerobic Dance Step Patterns

There are hundreds of possible step patterns that can be mixed in hundreds of different movement combinations. Many step patterns can be varied by changing the rhythm (slower or half time to faster or double time) or by changing a single movement (a knee lift) to a double movement (lifting the knee twice on each side). For added variety, a step pattern can travel from front to back, side to side, on a diagonal, or in a circle.

Remember that many step patterns can be modified to a high-, moderate-, or low-impact movement. For a high-impact movement, allow both feet to leave the floor. For a moderate-impact movement, keep one or both feet on the floor while fully extending the body upward, then lowering the heels to the floor. For a low-impact movement, keep one foot on the floor at all times and exaggerate the step pattern by vigorously lowering and lifting your body.

The following step patterns are examples of common movements used in aerobic dance.

Sample Step Patterns

STEP PATTERN: March [Figure 7.4 (a) and (b)].

Description: Alternately lift the knees up toward the chest.

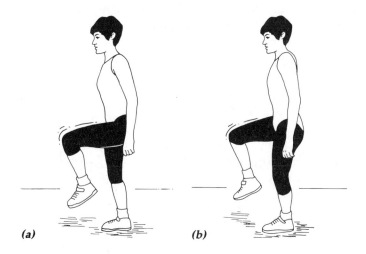

FIGURE 7.4
March sequence.

(a)   *(b)*

STEP PATTERN: Jog [Figure 7.5 (a) and (b)].

Description: Alternately lift the feet off the floor.

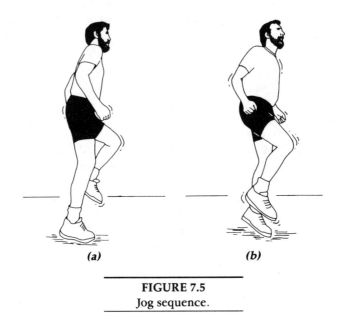

(a)   (b)

FIGURE 7.5
Jog sequence.

STEP PATTERN: Knee lift [Figure 7.6 (a) through (d)].

Description: Lift the right knee on count 1 and return the foot to the floor on count 2. Alternate right and left knees.

> **Variations:** The knee can be lifted to the side of the body.
> The intensity can be increased by adding a hop on count 2.
> The same knee can be lifted two or more consecutive times.

STEP PATTERN: Heel lift [Figure 7.7 (a) through (d)].

Description: Step to the right with the right foot on count 1, and lift the left heel up to the buttocks on count 2. Alternate from the right to the left side.

> **Variations:** The same heel can be lifted two or more consecutive times.
> This step can become a hopscotch by adding a jump onto both feet (feet apart) on count 1 and a hop during the heel lift on count 2.

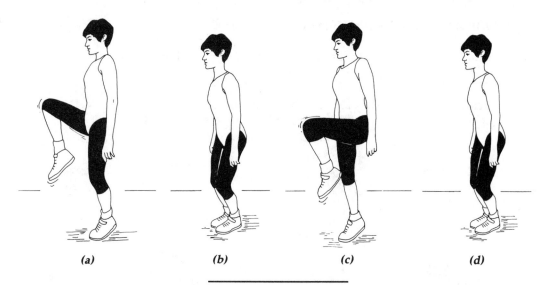

(a)   *(b)*   *(c)*   *(d)*

FIGURE 7.6
Knee lift sequence.

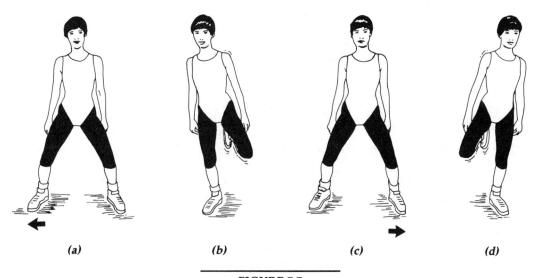

(a)   *(b)*   *(c)*   *(d)*

FIGURE 7.7
Heel lift sequence.

STEP PATTERN: Kick [Figure 7.8 (a) through (d)].

Description: Kick the right foot to the front on count 1 and return the foot to the floor on count 2. Alternate the right and left legs.

> **Variations:** Kick to the side or behind the body.
> To increase intensity, add a jump between kicks.
> The same foot can be kicked two or more consecutive times.

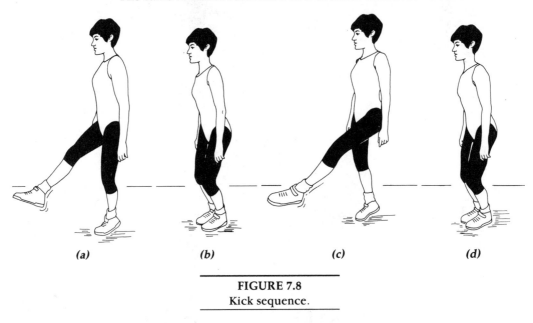

(a)   *(b)*   *(c)*   *(d)*

FIGURE 7.8
Kick sequence.

STEP PATTERN: Front heel [Figure 7.9 (a) through (d)].

Description: Place the heel of the right foot on the floor to the front on count 1, and return the foot next to the left foot on count 2. Alternate the right and left foot.

> **Variations:** To increase intensity, add a jump on count 2.
> The same heel can contact the floor two or more consecutive times.

STEP PATTERN: Step touch [Figure 7.10 (a) through (d)].

> **Variations:** Step to the right with the right foot on count 1, and cross the left heel on the floor in front of the right foot on count 2. The left foot is not weight-bearing, so the movement can be repeated to the left side.

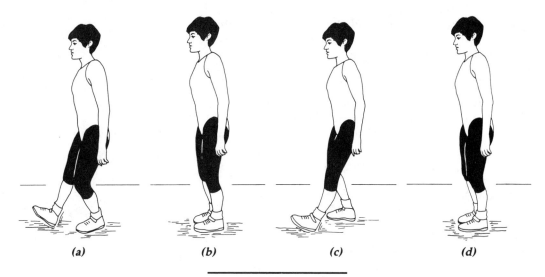

(a)   (b)   (c)   (d)

FIGURE 7.9
Front heel sequence.

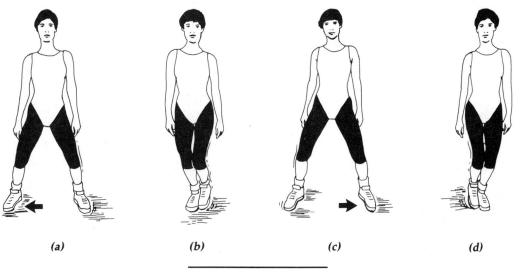

(a)   (b)   (c)   (d)

FIGURE 7.10
Step touch sequence.

STEP PATTERN: Step push [Figure 7.11 (a) through (d)].

Description: Step to the right with the right foot on count 1, and push the right foot back to the left foot on count 2. Alternate from the right to the left side.

> **Variations:** The same foot that steps to the side can step sideways two or more consecutive times.
> Step to the right and bounce or jump with the feet apart for 2 counts, then bounce or jump with the feet together for 2 counts. Repeat to the left.

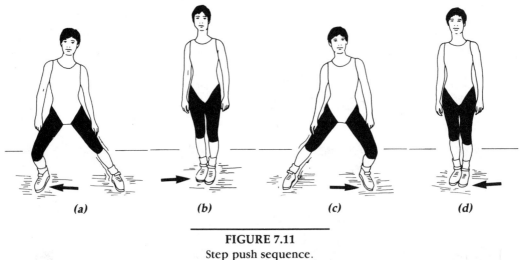

(a)   (b)   (c)   (d)

FIGURE 7.11
Step push sequence.

STEP PATTERN: Step point [Figure 7.12 (a) through (d)].

Description: Step to the right with the right foot on count 1, and raise up on the toes of the left foot on count 2. Alternate from the right to the left side.

STEP PATTERN: Twisting [Figure 7.13 (a) and (b)].

Description: Pivot on the balls of your feet from the right side to the left side, with the shoulders twisting in the opposite direction of the feet.

> **Variations:** A double twist can be performed by twisting and bouncing twice to the right, then repeating to the left.

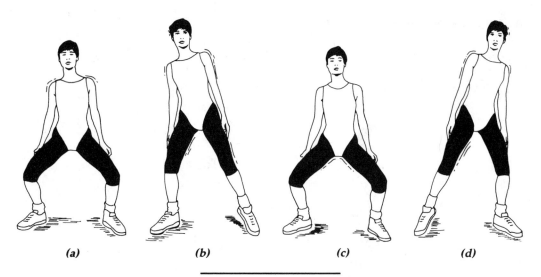

FIGURE 7.12
Step point sequence.

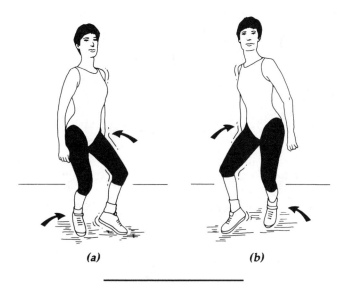

FIGURE 7.13
Twisting sequence.

STEP PATTERN: Jump [Figure 7.14 (a) and (b)].

Description: On count 1, push both feet off the floor and land on both feet.

    Variations: Jump and land on count 1, hold or bounce on count 2.

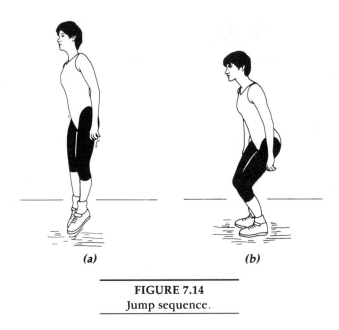

(a)   *(b)*

FIGURE 7.14
Jump sequence.

STEP PATTERN: Lunge [Figure 7.15 (a) through (d)].

Description: Turn to the right and place the left foot behind the right foot on count 1. Bring the feet back together on count 2. Alternate from the right to the left side.

    Variations: To increase intensity, add a jump on count 2.
                         The same foot can lunge back two or more consecutive times.

STEP PATTERN: Jumping jack [Figure 7.16 (a) and (b)].

Description: Spread the feet apart on count 1, and return the feet together on count 2. Be sure the knees are pointing over the center of the toes when the feet are apart.

    Variations: A double jumping jack can be performed by bouncing or jumping
                         with the feet apart for 2 counts and bouncing or jumping with the
                         feet together for 2 counts.

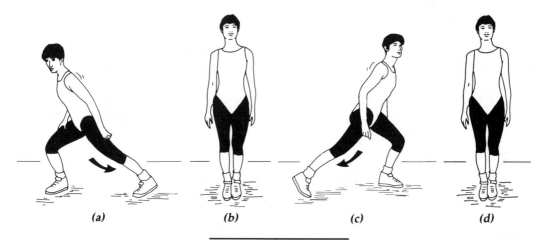

(a) (b) (c) (d)

FIGURE 7.15
Lunge sequence.

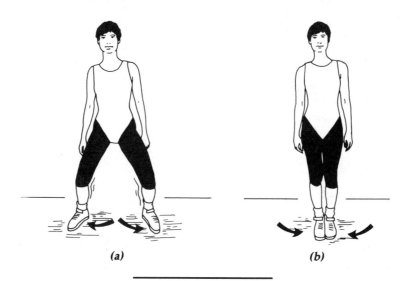

(a) (b)

FIGURE 7.16
Jumping jack sequence.

STEP PATTERN: Pendulum [Figure 7.17 (a) and (b)].

Description: Lift the right leg to the right side on count 1, and return it to the floor as you lift the left leg to the left side on count 2.

> **Variations:** A double pendulum can be performed by keeping the right leg extended to the right on count 2 while adding a hop on the left foot. Repeat to the left.

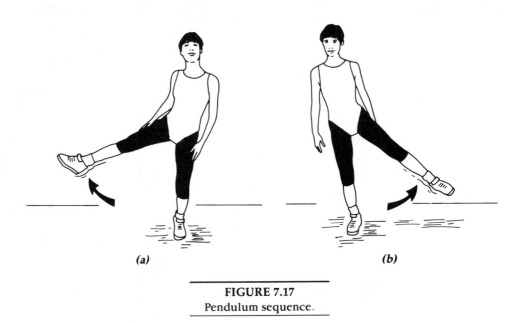

(a)   *(b)*

FIGURE 7.17
Pendulum sequence.

STEP PATTERN: Rocking horse [Figure 7.18 (a) and (b)].

Description: Start with one foot in front of the other. On count 1, lift the rear foot off the floor; on count 2, return the rear foot to the floor while lifting the front foot off the floor. Since the same leg is leading each time, be sure to change the foot that goes forward after eight or sixteen repetitions.

> **Variations:** A double rocking horse can be performed by keeping the front foot forward on count 2 while adding a hop on the supporting leg. Repeat to the rear.

STEP PATTERN: Grapevine [Figure 7.19 (a) through (d)].

Description: Step to the right with the right foot on count 1, cross the left foot in back of the right foot on count 2, step to the right with the right foot on count 3, and cross the left foot in front of the right foot on count 4. The last step is not weight-bearing, so the movement can be repeated to the left side.

> **Variations:** To increase intensity, add a jump on count 4.

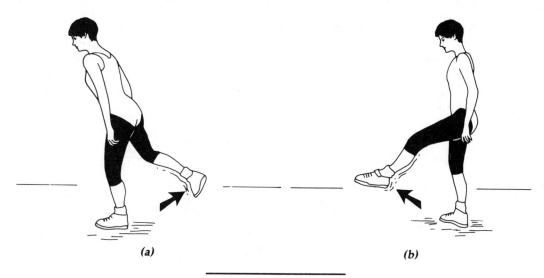

(a)   *(b)*

FIGURE 7.18
Rocking horse sequence.

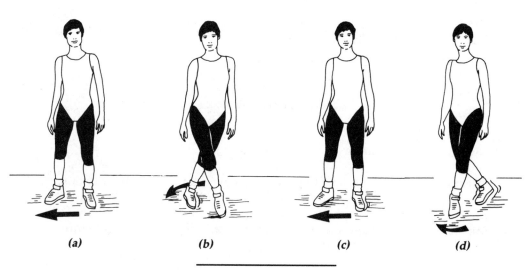

(a)   *(b)*   *(c)*   *(d)*

FIGURE 7.19
Grapevine sequence.

STEP PATTERN: Side stepping [Figure 7.20 (a) through (d)].

Description: Step to the right with the right foot on count 1, place the left foot next to the right foot on count 2, step to the right with the right foot on count 3, and touch the left foot next to the right foot. The last step is not weight-bearing, so it can repeat the movement to the left side.

Variations: To increase intensity, add a jump on count 4.

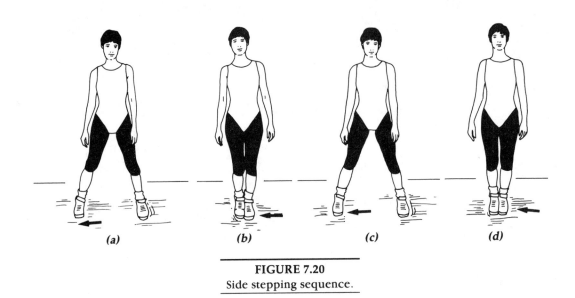

FIGURE 7.20
Side stepping sequence.

STEP PATTERN: Side leaps [Figure 7.21 (a) and (b)].

Description: Facing forward, leap to the right on the right foot while lifting the left leg to the left side on count 1. On count 2, land with both feet together. Repeat to the left.

Variations: Perform a series of consecutive leaps in one direction before leaping to the other side.

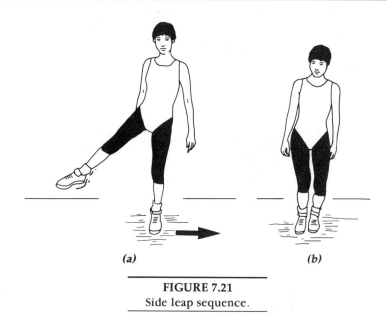

(a)   (b)

FIGURE 7.21
Side leap sequence.

Aerobic Dance Arm Movements

Once you have mastered the foot work, arms can be added to increase the exercise intensity and to enhance movement variety. Keep in mind that the activity from the arms can increase the energy cost of your aerobic exercise only by 20 to 25 percent. Therefore, try not to compromise the leg work by placing too much emphasis on the arm movements. In addition, be cautious of maintaining the arms at or above shoulder level for an extended period of time. Remember to vary among low-, mid-, and high-range arm movements frequently.

The following are sample arm movements that can be used to compliment your foot work.

Sample Arm Movements

ARM PATTERN: Clapping [Figure 7.22 (a) and (b)].

Description: Open the hands wide, then clap the hands together.

ARM PATTERN: Shoulder circles [Figure 7.23 (a) and (b)].

Description: Circle one or both shoulders forward or backward.

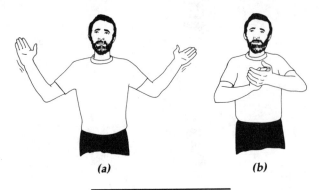

(a)   **(b)**

FIGURE 7.22
Clapping sequence.

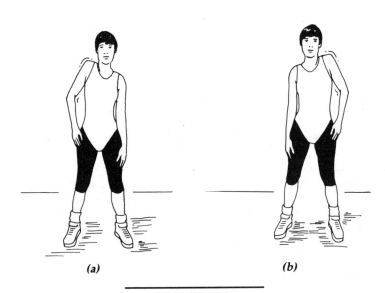

(a)   **(b)**

FIGURE 7.23
Alternating shoulder
circle sequence.

ARM PATTERN: Elbow circles [Figure 7.24 (a) and (b)].

Description: Circle one or both elbows forward or backward.

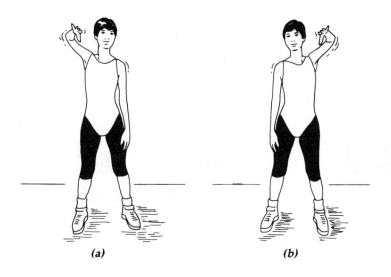

FIGURE 7.24
Alternating elbow circle
sequence.

(a)   (b)

ARM PATTERN: Arm circles [Figure 7.25 (a) and (b)].

Description: Circle one or both arms forward or backward.

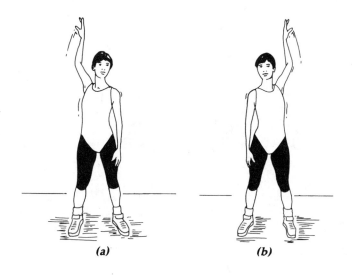

FIGURE 7.25
Alternating arm circle
sequence.

(a)   (b)

ARM PATTERN: Criss crosses [Figure 7.26 (a) through (d)].

Description: Cross the arms at waist or chest height. For each repetition, alternate the arm that crosses over the top.

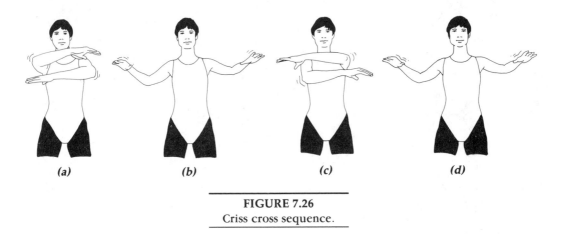

(a)   *(b)*   *(c)*   *(d)*

FIGURE 7.26
Criss cross sequence.

ARM PATTERN: Arm curls [Figure 7.27 (a) through (d)].

Description: With the elbows at the sides of the body, bring the hands up towards the shoulders and then down to the hips. The arms can move together or alternately.

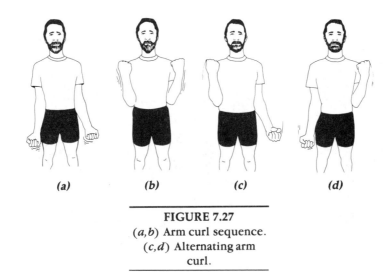

(a)   *(b)*   *(c)*   *(d)*

FIGURE 7.27
(*a,b*) Arm curl sequence.
(*c,d*) Alternating arm
curl.

ARM PATTERN: Press downs [Figure 7.28 (a) and (b)].

Description: Starting with the elbows at the sides of the body and the hands at the shoulders, press the hands down to the hips.

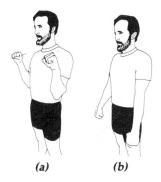

(a)   *(b)*

FIGURE 7.28
Press down sequence.

ARM PATTERN: Rowing [Figure 7.29 (a) through (d)].

Description: Extend the arms at chest height in front of the body. Pull both or one elbow straight back and then push forward.

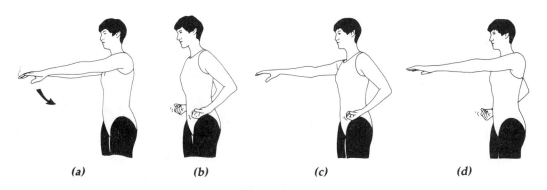

(a)   *(b)*   *(c)*   *(d)*

FIGURE 7.29
(*a,b*) Rowing sequence.
(*c,d*) Alternating rowing.

ARM PATTERN: Chest press [Figure 7.30 (a) through (d)].

Description: Start with the hands at chest level, elbows out to the side. Push the hands straight out and then back to the chest, either together or alternately.

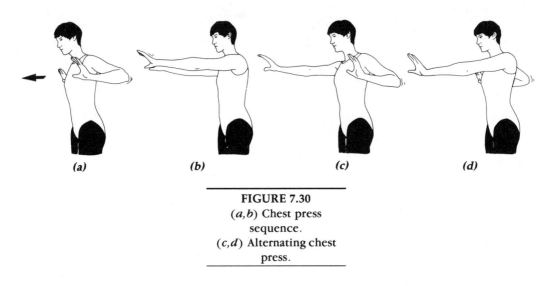

(a) (b) (c) (d)

FIGURE 7.30
(*a,b*) Chest press
sequence.
(*c,d*) Alternating chest
press.

ARM PATTERN: Punches [Figure 7.31 (a) through (d)].

Description: With one fist on the hips, punch the second fist on a low, middle, or high diagonal across the body. Alternate left and right fists.

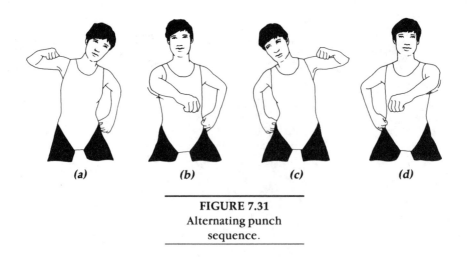

(a) (b) (c) (d)

FIGURE 7.31
Alternating punch
sequence.

ARM PATTERN: L position [Figure 7.32 (a) and (b)].

Description: Place one arm at shoulder height straight in front of the chest and the second arm at shoulder height straight out to the side. Swing the arms down to the waist and to the other side of the body.

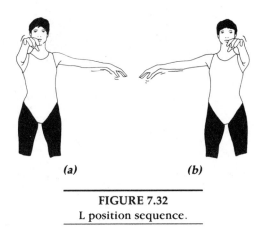

(a) *(b)*

FIGURE 7.32
L position sequence.

ARM PATTERN: Pendulum [Figure 7.33 (a) through (c)].

Description: Begin with both arms extended down and to one side of the body on a diagonal. Swing the arms down and then up to the other side of the body.

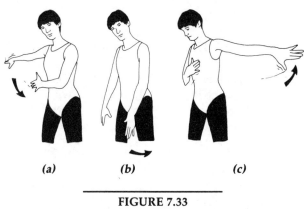

(a) *(b)* *(c)*

FIGURE 7.33
Pendulum sequence.

ARM PATTERN: Side press [Figure 7.34 (a) through (d)].

Description: Place both hands under the chin, elbows out to the side at shoulder height. Extend the arms straight out to the side and back under the chin either together or alternately.

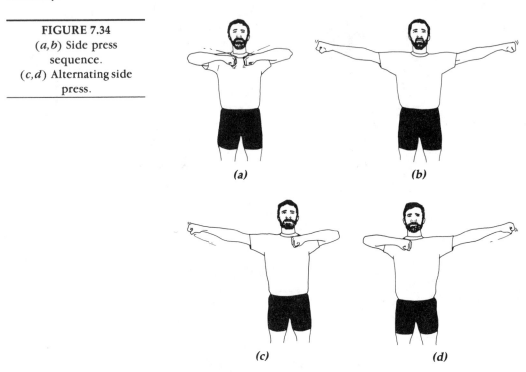

FIGURE 7.34
(*a,b*) Side press
sequence.
(*c,d*) Alternating side
press.

(a)   *(b)*

(c)   *(d)*

ARM PATTERN: Overhead press [Figure 7.35 (a) through (d)].

Description: Starting with the fingertips near the shoulders, elbows pointing down, press the arms to full extension above the head and then back down to the shoulder. Press both arms together or alternate the right and left arms.

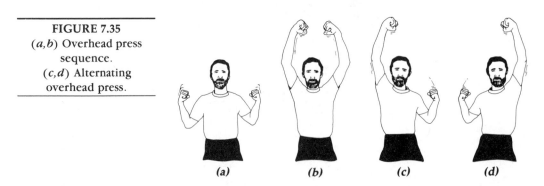

FIGURE 7.35
(*a,b*) Overhead press
sequence.
(*c,d*) Alternating
overhead press.

(a)   *(b)*   *(c)*   *(d)*

ARM PATTERN: Windmills [Figure 7.36 (a) through (d)].

Description: Starting with one arm straight down in front of the body and one arm straight up above the head, alternate arm position by swinging the arms back and forth.

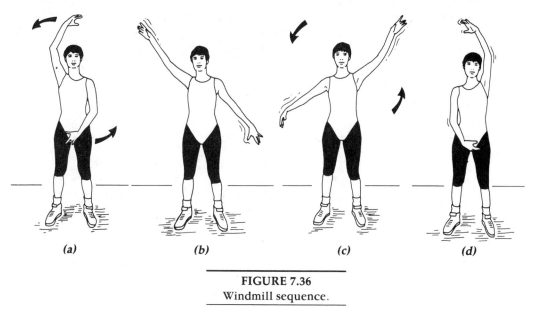

FIGURE 7.36
Windmill sequence.

ARM PATTERN: Full arm swings [Figure 7.37 (a) through (d)].

Description: Begin with both arms extended up over the head and on a diagonal. Swing the arms down in front of the body to the opposite diagonal.

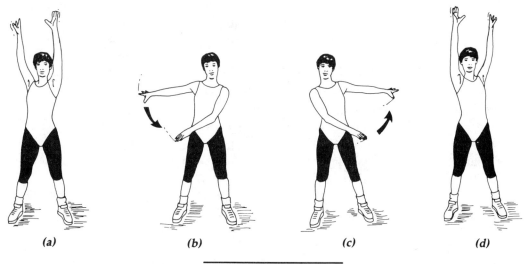

FIGURE 7.37
Full arm swing sequence.

Sample Aerobic Dance Routines

The following are examples of two aerobic dance routines. Routine 1 is easy to follow because it changes only one element at a time. In other words, each time a change is made in the choreography, only the footwork, the arm pattern, *or* the direction of movement changes. Routine 2 is made up of three combinations. A combination is a series of step patterns and arm movements combined and repeated in sequence several times in a row.

Routine 1

Sequence	Counts	Direction	Step Pattern	Arm Movement
1	8	In place	March or jog	No arms
2	8	In place	March or jog	4 alternating arm curls
3	8	Forward	March or jog	4 alternating arm curls
4	8	Backward	March or jog	4 alternating arm curls

Repeat sequence 3 and 4

Repeat sequence 2

5	8	In place	4 front heels	4 alternating arm curls
6	8	In place	4 front heels	4 L positions

Repeat sequence 6

7	8	In place	4 kicks	4 L positions
8	8	In place	4 kicks	4 claps
9	8	Forward	4 kicks	4 claps
10	8	Backward	4 kicks	4 claps

Repeat sequence 9 and 10

Repeat sequence 8

11	8	In place	4 knee lifts	4 claps
12	8	In place	4 knee lifts	4 criss crosses
13	8	Forward	4 knee lifts	4 criss crosses
14	8	Backward	4 knee lifts	4 criss crosses

Repeat sequence 13 and 14, changing the arms to 4 press downs

Repeat sequence 12, with 4 press downs

15	8	In place	4 step pushes	4 press downs
16	8	In place	4 step pushes	4 side presses

Repeat sequence 16, changing the arms to 4 press downs

17	8	In place	4 lunges	4 press downs
18	8	In place	4 lunges	4 single arm punches

Repeat sequence 18 two more times

Routine 2

Sequence	Counts	Direction	Step Pattern	Arm Movements
1	8	Forward	4 knee lifts	4 overhead presses
2	8	In place	4 step pushes	4 side presses
3	8	Backward	4 kicks	4 chest presses
4	8	In place	4 lunges	4 press downs

Repeat sequence 1–4 two more times

Sequence	Counts	Direction	Step Pattern	Arm Movements
5	8	To the right	4 side leaps	4 overhead presses
6	8	In place	4 front heels	4 L positions
7	8	To the left	4 side leaps	4 overhead presses
8	8	In place	4 front heels	4 L positions

Repeat sequence 5–8 two more times

Sequence	Counts	Direction	Step Pattern	Arm Movements
9	8	Forward	Jog	4 alternating arm curls
10	8	In place	Twist	4 alternating side presses
11	8	Backward	4 jumping jacks	4 claps
12	8	In place	Step point	4 full arm swings

Repeat sequence 9–12 two more times

Cooling Down after Aerobic Exercise

Cooling down after aerobic exercise is extremely important. You should never stop moving immediately following vigorous exercise. During aerobic activity, large quantities of blood are pumped to the working muscles. If you suddenly stop all movement, the blood pools in the legs because the muscles are no longer contracting to help return the extra blood. You may become dizzy or light-headed and may even feel faint.

A cool-down period also reduces the risk of cardiac complications by allowing the heart rate to gradually return to normal. In addition, a cool-down promotes faster removal of metabolic waste products, thus resulting in less muscle soreness.

Do not sit or lie down on the floor until your heart rate has slowed down to 120 beats per minute or lower. After completing the aerobic segment of your class, continue to move slowly, using movement patterns such as step touches and step points along with gentle arm swings.

Circuit and Interval Training

So far we have discussed continuous exercise as a way of improving aerobic fitness. It is also possible to increase cardiovascular endurance using intermittent exercise techniques. Two popular alternative methods used in aerobic dance classes are circuit training and interval training.

Circuit Training

Circuit training involves exercising continuously at a series of exercise stations, each with a specific fitness objective. The major purpose of circuit training is to improve a number of fitness components in one exercise session. For example, a circuit might be designed to improve cardiovascular endurance and muscular strength.

Most circuits are designed with ten to twenty stations. Each station is posted with a sign that indicates the task to be completed. An equal number of participants perform the assigned task at each station for a specified time (usually between thirty seconds and two minutes). On command, participants move clockwise or counterclockwise to the next station. The entire circuit can be repeated two to three times.

Many circuits alternate strength and aerobic stations throughout the exercise room (see Model 1), although some circuits are designed with strength training stations around the perimeter of the room and one aerobic station in the center (see Model 2). When using Model 2, participants exercise together during the aerobic portion and split into groups to work at each of the strength stations.

To prevent a significant drop in exercise heart rate, it is important that the aerobic activity is not interrupted by long periods of nonaerobic work such as strength training. When using Model 1, it is best to group several aerobic stations in a row followed by one strength station. For example, three consecutive aerobic stations at thirty seconds each will provide one and one-half minutes of vigorous exercise, and one strength station will provide thirty seconds of resistance work. For Model 2, more time can be devoted to the aerobic station performed in unison (three to four minutes) than the strength stations performed in groups (thirty to forty-five seconds).

Model 1

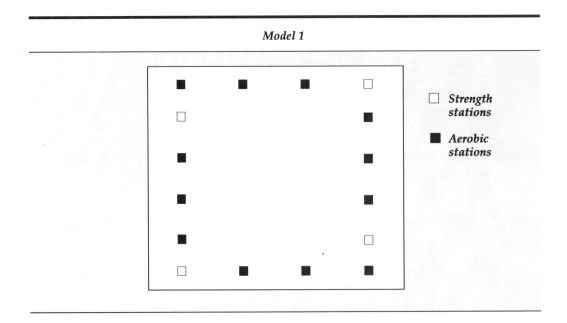

☐ *Strength stations*

■ *Aerobic stations*

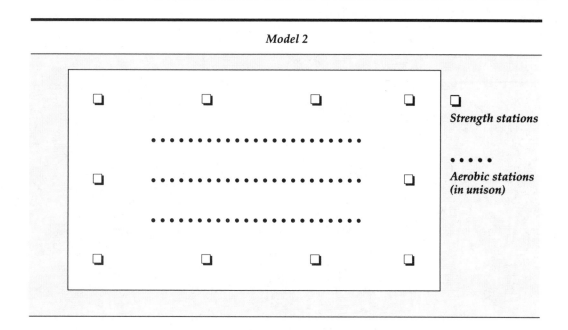

Typical movements for the aerobic dance stations include such exercises as knee lifts, lunges, jumping jacks, and jogging. Strength stations usually incorporate some form of resistance using light weights or bands to strengthen specific muscles of the trunk, arms, and legs. Table 7.1 presents an example of a Model 1–type circuit that targets strength and aerobic fitness.

Interval Training

For the more advanced aerobic dancer, interval training is a difficult and challenging technique that not only improves aerobic fitness but also enhances the capacity for anaerobic exercise. Anaerobic training is useful for performing intense activity over very short periods of time. Interval training involves high-intensity work bouts at near-maximal heart rate followed by active rest or recovery periods. Because participants work at very high intensities, the rest phase is necessary to recover from vigorous exercise and to prepare for the next exercise interval.

Table 7.1 Circuit Training Model

Type of circuit: Cardiovascular/strength
Number of stations: 12
Time per station: 30 seconds
Number of times through circuit: 3
Total time: 18 minutes (Time per station × Number of stations × Number of times through circuit)

Stations	First and Third Time through Circuit	Second Time through Circuit
1. Jog	Feet low	Knees high to the front
2. Kicks	Front kicks	Side kicks
3. Front heels	Low impact	High impact
4. Elbow press with bands	Step touch	Step point
5. Rocking horse	Doubles	Singles
6. Knee lift	Doubles	Singles
7. Hopscotch	Low impact	High impact
8. Lat pull down with bands	Step heel	Step point
9. Pendulum	Doubles	Singles
10. Jumping jacks	Doubles	Singles
11. Lunge	Low impact	High impact
12. Chest cross with bands	Step touch	Step point

Exercising at near-maximal heart rate produces metabolic waste products that accumulate in the muscle, causing pain and discomfort. When using this advanced technique, you must be highly motivated to exercise as hard as you possibly can during the exercise bouts.

Typically, exercise and rest intervals vary from thirty seconds to three minutes in length and are repeated eight to twenty times during the aerobic segment of the class. The recovery intervals are usually twice as long as the exercise bouts. For example, exercise intervals of one minute would be followed by recovery periods of approximately two minutes.

High-impact movements such as jumps and runs are choreographed to fast-paced music during the work bouts to produce high heart rates. During the active rest period, moderately paced movements such as walking and step touches are performed. Keep in mind that if you have enough energy left during the active rest phase to continue moving at a vigorous pace, you did not work hard enough during the exercise bout. Table 7.2 presents an example of an interval training session.

Table 7.2 Sample Interval Training Session

Number of intervals: 12
Length of exercise bouts: 1 minute
Length of active rest bouts: 2 minutes
Music tempo for exercise bouts: 160 beats per minute or more
Music tempo for active rest bouts: Around 120 beats per minute
Total time: 36 minutes [(Length of exercise bout + Length of active rest bout) × Number of intervals]

Exercise Bout #1, #4, #7, and #10
A. Jog with knees high to front—16 counts
B. Jumping jacks—16 counts
C. Single pendulums—16 counts
Repeat A, B, and C until 1 minute is completed.

Active Rest Bout #1, #4, #7, and #10
A. Step touch in place—16 counts
B. Step touch forward 8 counts and backward 8 counts—repeat 4 times
C. Step point in place—16 counts
D. Step point forward 8 counts and backward 8 counts—repeat 4 times
E. Step heel in place—16 counts
F. Step heel forward 8 counts and backward 8 counts—repeat 4 times
Repeat A through F until 2 minutes are completed.

Exercise Bout #2, #5, #8, and #11
A. Kick forward—16 counts
B. Knee lifts in place—16 counts
C. Jumping jack backward—16 counts
D. High jumps (4 counts each) in place—16 counts
Repeat A, B, C, and D until 1 minute is completed.

Active Rest Bout #2, #5, #8, and #11
A. Step point in place—16 counts
B. Step heel in place—16 counts
C. Step point forward—8 counts
D. Step heel backward—8 counts
Repeat C and D until 2 minutes are completed.

Exercise Bout #3, # 6, #9, and #12
A. Single pendulums in place—16 counts
B. Single rocking horses, right leg forward—16 counts
C. Twist in place—16 counts
D. Single rocking horses, left leg forward—16 counts
E. Twist in place—16 counts
Repeat A through E until 1 minute is completed.

Active Rest Bout # 3, #6, #9, and #12
A. Knee lifts in place—16 counts
B. Heel lifts in place—16 counts
C. Knee lifts forward—16 counts
D. Heel lifts backward—16 counts
Repeat C and D until 2 minutes are completed.

KEY POINTS IN CHAPTER 7

1. Aerobic dance movements can be performed using high-, moderate-, or low-impact step patterns.

2. It is important to select or modify the amount of impact according to your personal needs.

3. To enhance performance and reduce the risk of injury, always warm up and stretch before aerobic activity.

4. Perform all aerobic dance movements using proper body alignment and avoid potentially hazardous movements.

5. To prevent pooling of blood in the legs and to reduce the risk of cardiac complications, always cool down after aerobic activity.

6. Circuit training involves exercising continuously at a series of exercise stations, each with a specific fitness objective. Most aerobic dance circuits emphasize muscular strength and cardiovascular endurance.

7. Interval training is an advanced technique that uses high-intensity work bouts at near-maximal heart rate followed by active rest or recovery periods. Interval training enhances both aerobic and anaerobic fitness.

8 *Weight Management*

TEST YOUR KNOWLEDGE

Answer true or false to the following statements:

1. The average weight of the American population is increasing.   True   False

   Answer: True. Even though Americans are obsessed with weight loss, the population continues to get fatter.

2. The best way to measure fat loss is to periodically weigh yourself on a bathroom scale.   True   False

   Answer: False. A scale can only indicate a change in weight. It cannot distinguish between changes in fat, water, or muscle weight.

3. A significant drop in calories will effectively reduce your percentage of body fat.   True   False

   Answer: False. Your body will think it is being starved and will hold on to its fat stores for emergency use.

4. Dieting is more effective for losing weight than exercising.   True   False

   Answer: False. A combination of sensible dieting and moderate exercise is more effective than either diet or exercise alone.

Dieting

Each year, new diet books rise to the top of the best-seller list, tempting millions of overweight individuals with the latest fads in weight loss. Oddly enough, epidemic dieting is not confined to the truly overweight. Many people who are considered to be at a healthy weight will diet for fear of becoming fat.

Whether a weight problem is real or imagined, people continue their search for the ultimate gimmick that will shed those unwanted pounds forever! Desiring the "perfect" body, men and women will buy powders, potions, and devices that promise to melt, shock, roll, squeeze, or vibrate the fat away. They will suffer through countless diets, such as the grapefruit diet, the fasting diet, and the high-protein diet. Some will even resort to plastic surgery to reshape their appearances. Unfortunately, few diets will result in permanent fat loss, and even fewer weight-loss devices will produce the desired results.

Although American society is obsessed with weight loss, the average weight of the population continues to increase. Are overweight people destined to remain fat? Only if they continue to rely on weight-loss gimmicks rather than commonsense nutritional and exercise practices.

Body Types

Have you ever wondered why some people have great muscle definition and rarely lift weights, or why some people are thin and never exercise or diet? Muscle definition seems to come easily for some and fat appears to quickly melt off others. Many of these characteristics are genetic and can be attributed to a person's particular body type. Although you can improve your appearance through diet and exercise, you cannot change your basic body type (short of having surgery). Body type is determined by the way in which fat is distributed on your body, the extent of your muscle definition and development, the length of your limbs, and the shape of your skeletal system.

There are three basic body types. Although your body may not fit all the characteristics of one type, you will probably find that you have more qualities of one type than another. It is also possible that you may be a combination of two body types.

The following descriptions and diagrams will help you to determine your body type:

Ectomorph: Characterized by a long rectangular shape, narrow hips, small waist, small bones, long limbs, and a low total amount of body fat (Figure 8.1).

Endomorph: Characterized by a round, soft shape, small to medium bones, fat around the hips and thighs, lack of muscle definition, and a high fat-to-muscle ratio on trunk and limbs (Figure 8.2).

Mesomorph: Characterized by a square shape with broad shoulders and hips, narrow waist, well-defined muscles on trunk and hips, a high muscle-to-fat ratio, and medium to large bones (Figure 8.3).

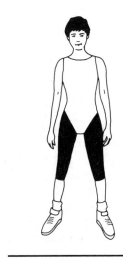

FIGURE 8.1
Ectomorph.

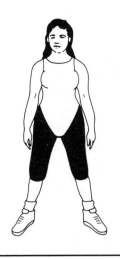

FIGURE 8.2
Endomorph.

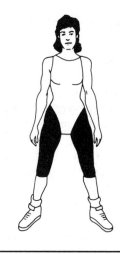

FIGURE 8.3
Mesomorph.

Understanding your body type will help you set realistic exercise and nutritional goals. For example, if you are extremely muscular and large boned, you will never resemble a thin fashion model no matter how much dieting you do. Similarly, if you have long limbs and a small musculoskeletal frame, you are not likely to look like a body builder regardless of the amount of strength training you perform. Although exercise and diet cannot change a pear-shaped body into an hourglass figure, exercise and diet can certainly change a large pear into a smaller pear.

Body Composition

Body composition refers to your percentage of body fat and lean body weight. Your lean body weight consists of your muscles, bones, nervous system tissue, skin, and organs. Your fat weight includes essential body fat necessary for maintenance of life and reproduction and nonessential or excess fat. Ideally, healthy men's bodies should be around 8 to 15 percent body fat whereas healthy women's bodies should be around 15 to 22 percent body fat. Unfortunately, the average middle-aged American male has 23 percent body fat and the average middle-aged American female has 32 percent.

The higher the percentage of body fat, the greater the risk of developing cardiovascular disease. In addition, extremely heavy people place excessive stress on their musculoskeletal system, increasing their risk for sustaining injuries. A combination of sensible eating and moderate exercise is the safest and most effective method for reducing the percentage of body fat.

Measuring Body Fat

The bathroom scale is the most common method used to measure body weight. Unfortunately, the scale cannot differentiate between body fat and lean body weight. In fact, the scale cannot distinguish between the weight of your muscles and that of body fluids. When your weight naturally fluctuates between two and four pounds a day on a scale, you have no way of knowing what caused the increase or decrease in your weight. It is certain, however, that you have not lost four pounds of fat in a twenty-four-hour period, since you must burn 3,500 calories to lose one pound of fat. A vigorous thirty-minute aerobic dance session will burn approximately 230 calories. A bathroom scale is, therefore, a poor method for measuring changes in your fat weight.

The most accurate methods for measuring body fat are underwater weighing, skinfold measures, and electrical impedance. These methods are not practical for most people, however, because they require sophisticated instruments and a technician to administer the tests.

The most practical methods for measuring fat loss are the pinch test, your mirror, and the fit of your clothes. Although these tests can be subjective, they are more accurate than using a bathroom scale to measure fat loss.

To perform the pinch test, pinch the skin and fat at your waist just above the hip and measure the thickness of the pinch with a ruler (Figure 8.4). More than an inch for men and an inch and a half for women would be considered too much fat. A passing score would be less than half an inch for men and less than one inch for women.

Another method for measuring body fat is your mirror. The mirror rarely lies. Wearing as few clothes as possible, observe yourself in a mirror (preferably full length). Look for large fat deposits. Repeat this process periodically, looking for changes in the size of your fat deposits.

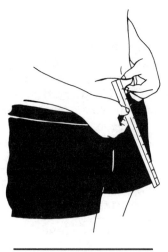

FIGURE 8.4
Pinch test.

Finally, a decrease in your clothing size is a sure sign of changes in your body composition. As you begin to exercise, your muscles become firmer and your body fat decreases, resulting in a loss of inches. Subsequently, you'll notice that your clothes have become looser.

A note of caution should be added. Exercising while wearing impermeable clothing or sitting in a sauna are common ways to attempt to lose weight. Although these techniques result in a weight change on the scale, the vast majority of the loss is water. These methods have no effect on fat. In addition, losing large amounts of water can cause dehydration and can be hazardous to your health.

Effective Techniques for Weight Management

Research shows that the most effective method for weight control is a moderate reduction in caloric intake and participation in a regular exercise program.

To reduce your weight through diet, here are some nutritional recommendations to follow:

1. Reduce the amount of fat consumed in your diet. Trim extra fat from your meat and use smaller quantities of high-fat foods such as salad dressing, butter, or margarine.

2. Reduce the amount of sugar in your diet. Sugary products tend to be high in calories and have little nutritional value.

3. Eat plenty of complex carbohydrates such as whole-grain breads, pastas, cereals, and vegetables. These foods provide much-needed fiber (as do fruits), are a good source of vitamins and minerals, and are generally low in calories.

4. Do not fast or drastically lower your caloric intake. When your body thinks that it is in a state of starvation, it protects itself by retaining body fat. It becomes increasingly more difficult to shed unwanted fat if you drastically reduce your caloric intake frequently.

To reduce your weight through exercise, follow these activity guidelines:

1. Exercise at moderate intensities for longer durations. Since lower exercise intensities allow you to perform aerobic dance for longer periods, you will probably burn more calories than if you were to perform high-intensity exercise for a short duration. In addition, lower exercise intensities reduce the risk of musculoskeletal injury.

2. Start gradually. If you progress too quickly and get hurt, you will lose the weight-loss benefits of exercise while you are nursing your injury.

3. Become more physically active throughout the day. Take the stairs instead of the elevator or if possible walk or ride a bike to work or school instead of driving.

KEY POINTS IN CHAPTER 8

1. Although American society is obsessed with weight loss, the population continues to get fatter.

2. The percentage of body fat for the average middle-aged American is classified as "unhealthy," because it is too high.

3. The higher the percentage of body fat, the greater the risk for developing cardiovascular disease and musculoskeletal injury.

4. The bathroom scale is most frequently used to measure changes in body weight, but it is a poor measure of fat loss.

5. Although the most accurate laboratory procedures for measuring body fat are underwater weighing, skinfold measures, and electrical impedance, the most practical home techniques for measuring fat loss are the pinch test, the mirror, and the fit of your clothes.

6. The most effective method for weight control is a moderate reduction in caloric intake and participation in a regular exercise program.

9 *Aerobic Dance Injuries*

TEST YOUR KNOWLEDGE

Answer true or false to the following statements:

1. If you have a minor pain while doing aerobic dance, you should continue to exercise, because the injury will soon heal and you do not want to lose any of the benefits you have already gained from your exercise program.   True   False

   Answer: False. A minor injury can become serious if it is not properly rested and treated.

2. Overuse injuries such as shin splints occur gradually and usually without a history of a specific incident triggering the injury.   True   False

   Answer: True. Repeated and excessive mechanical stress on a specific area of the body can result in overuse injuries such as shin splints.

3. The best treatment for swelling is to place heat on the afflicted area.   True   False

   Answer: False. Ice is more effective than heat for reducing swelling.

4. If you are suffering from swelling, restricted movement in a joint, or pain and discomfort, you should ask your instructor for the best form of treatment that you can administer at home.   True   False

   Answer: False. You should discontinue exercise and seek medical attention.

Overuse Injuries

The most common form of aerobic dance injuries are overuse injuries, which are caused by repeated and excessive mechanical stress on a specific area of the body. Most forms of vigorous exercise place a certain amount of stress on the musculoskeletal system. Given enough time to adapt to the increased stresses of exercise, your bones, muscles, tendons, and ligaments become stronger and more resilient. If you rush the process, however, you are more likely to suffer an overuse injury.

Overuse injuries happen gradually, often without being triggered by a specific incident. Sufferers of such injuries experience physical discomfort and sometimes swelling and limited range of joint motion. If a person continues to exercise while in pain, the injury will become much more severe, limiting participation in any form of activity. For example, a common overuse injury among aerobic dancers is mild shin pain. If not properly treated, mild shin pain could develop into a more serious stress fracture.

To reduce the risk of overuse injuries, you must try to minimize the amount of mechanical stress placed on your body. The following are guidelines for decreasing the risk of developing overuse injuries:

1. Begin exercising in a class that is appropriate for your present level of physical fitness. Injuries often occur when individuals exercise at a level that is too advanced for their present skills.

2. Progress slowly. Even the most physically fit individual can get hurt by abruptly increasing the exercise workload without allowing the musculoskeletal system time to adapt.

3. Make only one change at a time. If you decide to increase your exercise frequency by attending one more aerobic dance class per week, do not simultaneously increase the amount of aerobic activity in each exercise session. Your body must be allowed to gradually adjust to the increased demands of each new change.

4. Optimize intensity, duration, and frequency of exercise. As the intensity, duration, and frequency of your aerobic dance sessions increase, so do your risks for sustaining musculoskeletal injury.

5. Select appropriate shoes and aerobic dance floors. Shoes and floors with adequate stability, shock absorption, and traction will minimize your risk of injury.

6. Do not perform hazardous exercises, such as deep knee bends or unsupported forward flexion in a standing position. Become familiar with risky exercises so that you know which ones to avoid.

7. Listen to your body. You will soon learn to recognize the difference between mild discomfort and pain. Pain is the body's way of warning you that something is wrong. Mild muscle soreness following vigorous exercise is to be expected. However, pain in any of your joints or bones indicates a problem. Discontinue exercises that cause you unusual discomfort, and consult your physician to determine the cause of the pain.

Treating Injuries

If you are suffering from swelling, restricted joint range of movement, or pain and discomfort, seek medical attention before you return to exercise.

RICE (Rest, Ice, Compression, and Elevation) is the most common treatment recommended by physicians for soft tissue injuries. *R*est minimizes the stress placed on the injured area, while *I*ce, *C*ompression, and *E*levation all help to control swelling. Swelling results from bleeding or inflammation in and around the injured area, which causes pain and restricts movement.

Common Aerobic Dance Injuries

Any pain or discomfort that does not improve with rest should be treated by a medical practitioner. Remember that an insignificant injury can become very serious if it is ignored and you continue to exercise.

Although medical practitioners should always be the ones to diagnose your injury and prescribe the appropriate treatment, Table 9.1 will familiarize you with the symptoms of common aerobic dance injuries and their probable causes.

Table 9.1   Common Aerobic Dance Injuries

Name of Injury	Description of Injury	Symptoms	Possible Cause of Injury
Ankle Sprain	Overstretching or tearing of a ligament	Sharp pain around the joint; probable swelling	Too much traction between shoes and surface
Bursitis	Irritation of a bursa (fluid-filled sac located where friction might occur in the body)	Pain and stiffness in the area of the bursa	Constant pressure on the bursa from weight-bearing activities
Lower Back Pain	Sprain or strain of lower back; pressure on nerves	Muscles of lower back may go into spasm; sharp pain in lower back or radiating to other areas	Congenital abnormality; poor body mechanics; poor posture; poor exercise technique

Table 9.1 – Continued

Name of Injury	Description of Injury	Symptoms	Possible Cause of Injury
Metatar-salgia (Foot)	Bruising of the joints in the ball of the foot	Pain in the ball of the foot	Extreme repeated impacts on the ball of the foot
Muscle Strain	Overstretching or tearing of a muscle or tendon	Muscle tenderness; possible swelling	Poor flexibility; sudden violent contraction of a muscle
Neuroma (Foot)	An entrapment of part of a nerve, usually between the third and fourth toe	Sharp radiating pain to the ends of the toes	Narrow-fitting shoes
Patello-Femoral Pain Syndrome (Knee)	The knee cap does not pull through normal alignment: may result in gradual degener-ation of the cartilage that lines the back of the knee cap (chondromalacia)	Pain around or under the knee cap; may feel or hear a grinding noise	Poor body mechanics; abnormal position of the knee cap; excessive flexion and extension of the knee with heavy resistance; excessive pronation (supporting the weight on the inside borders of the feet)
Plantar Fasciitis (Foot)	Inflammation of the band that runs the length of the sole of the foot	Pain and tightening along the length of the arch of the foot	Stressful weight-bearing activities with an inability to effectively absorb shock

Table 9.1—Continued

Name of Injury	Description of Injury	Symptoms	Possible Cause of Injury
Shin Splints	Can be a number of conditions, including microtears in the muscle tissue or stress fractures in the tibia	Pain and tenderness in the shin region	Poor shoes; fallen arches; exercising on unyielding surfaces; poor body mechanics
Stress Fracture	Beginning of a bone fracture	Sharp pain in the bone	Stressful weight-bearing activities with an inability to effectively absorb shock
Tendinitis	Inflammation of a tendon	Pain over the tendon	Improper warm-up; repeated forceful stretching; poor shoes and floors

KEY POINTS IN CHAPTER 9

1. The most common type of aerobic dance injury is caused by repeated and excessive mechanical stress on specific areas of the body.

2. To minimize overuse injuries, progress slowly; optimize intensity, duration, and frequency of exercise; select appropriate aerobic dance shoes and exercise surfaces; and avoid hazardous exercise techniques.

3. Discontinue any physical activity that causes excessive discomfort and pain. Remember, pain is the body's way of warning you that something is wrong.

4. Any pain or discomfort that does not improve with rest should be seen by a medical practitioner.

Index

Big Band™

Size	12" × 1/2"	12" × 3/4"	16" × 1/2"	16" × 3/4"
Quantity	$	$	$	$
1-9	2.00	2.50	2.75	3.00
10-49	1.00	1.25	1.35	1.50
50-99	.90	1.10	1.25	1.35
100-249	.80	1.00	1.15	1.25
250-499	.70	.90	1.05	1.15
500-999	.65	.85	1.00	1.10
1000+	.60	.80	.95	1.05

For more Information on SPRI's line of rubber resistive exercise products, to request a catalog, or to place an order, call SPRI Products, Inc., toll-free at 1–800–222–7774.